SURF FLEX

FLEXIBILITY, YOGA, AND CONDITIONING FOR THE ULTIMATE SURFING EXPERIENCE!

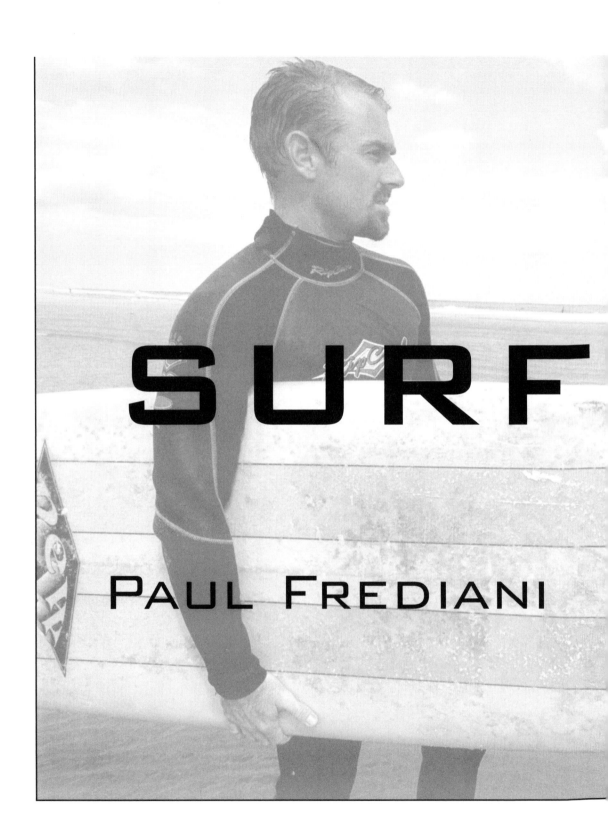

SURF

PAUL FREDIANI

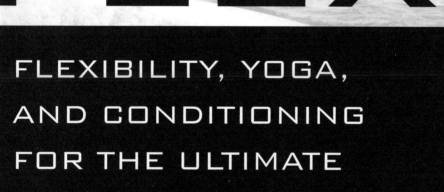

FLEX

FLEXIBILITY, YOGA, AND CONDITIONING FOR THE ULTIMATE SURFING EXPERIENCE!

PHOTOGRAPHY BY PETER FIELD PECK

Hatherleigh Press • New York, New York

A GETFITNOW.COM BOOK

SURF FLEX: FLEXIBILITY, YOGA, AND CONDITIONING FOR THE ULTIMATE SURFING EXPERIENCE

A Getfitnow.com Book

Text Copyright © 2001 by Paul Frediani
Photographs Copyright © 2001 The Hatherleigh Company, Ltd.

Hatherleigh Press/Getfitnow.com Books
An Affiliate of W.W. Norton & Company, Inc.
522 46th Avenue Suite 200
Long Island City, NY 11101
1-800-528-2550
Visit our website: www.getfitnow.com

> **DISCLAIMER:** Before beginning any exercise program consult your physician. The authors and publisher of this book and workout disclaim any liability, personal or professional, resulting from the misapplication of any of the training procedures described in this publication.

All Getfitnow.com titles are available for bulk purchase, special promotions, and premiums. For more information, please contact the manager of our Special Sales Department at 1-800-528-2550.

Library of Congress Cataloging-in-Publication Data

Frediani, Paul, 1952–
     Surf flex : flexibility, yoga, and conditioning for the ultimate surfing experience /
     Paul Frediani
         p.   cm.
     ISBN 1-57826-078-7 (alk. paper)
     1. Surfing—Training.   2. Exercise.   3. Yoga   I. Title.
     GV840.S8 F72 2000
     613.7'16—dc21   00-040877
                                                                           CIP

Cover design by Lisa Fyfe
Text design and composition by John Reinhardt Book Design
Principle photography by Peter Field Peck with Canon® cameras and lenses on Fuji® print film

On the cover:

Chris Curry rides to victory. Encuentro 2000. Dominican Republic. Photo by Chad Oakly.

Printed on acid-free paper   10 9 8 7 6 5 4

I'd like to dedicate this book to

My son Paolo,
the heart that beats outside my chest.

My brother Enrico,
who would be the world champion if the best surfer
were the one having the most fun.

My grandfather Enrico Gemignani,
a patriot, adventurer, and sailor whose love of the
sea runs through our veins.

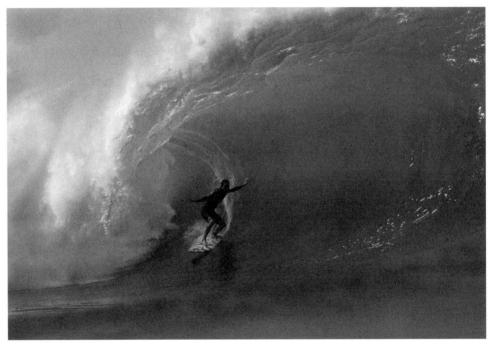

GERRY LOPEZ IN THE TUBE. PHOTO COURTESY CARBAJAL DESIGNS.

ACKNOWLEDGMENTS

My associate Stew Smith told me that when he was training to be a Navy SEAL, in one exercise, the SEALs had their goggles blackened and were told to jump off the ship and attempt to swim in a straight line. Inevitably, they would all swim in a big circle and back to the vessel. They did so because the dominant side of their bodies would always pull them in that direction.

This was the feeling I had as I began writing *Surf Flex*: a strong sense of going back home and of trying to give back something to the surfers past, present, and future. Nothing gives me more joy in my life than going out surfing with my son and brother...surfing to a point of exhaustion then going to the nearest Mexican restaurant, chowing down, and lying to each other about how big the waves were and how many times we got tubed. I also want to stay healthy and keep surfing with them until the Big Man taps me on the shoulder and tells me to dry off.

There are many people I'd like to thank for helping me with this book: my publisher, Andrew Flach, who had the foresight and courage to publish *Surf Flex*; my editor, Heather Ogilvie, who deserves all the credit for making sense of my chicken scratch and my waterlogged

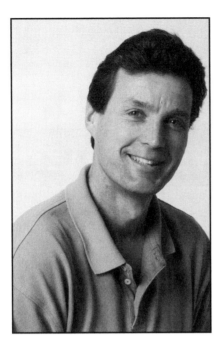

brain; Peter Peck, for the beautiful photography; Paul West, director of the U.S. Surf Team; all the fine surfers on the team for allowing me to put them through the workouts; the cool and talented Dominican Republic Surf Team; Stew Smith, truly an officer and gentleman; Renee Meier, the cornerstone of my life; all the surfers who took the time to contribute; and the models who grace these pages: Clay Bennett (surfboard designer for Ozboards and winner of over 500 trophies as an amateur and professional surfer), Marian Hunter, Yancy Spencer IV, Missie Haefer, Nastassja Gwizdak, Derek Wiltison, Tracy O'Mahony, Marilyn Austin, Aja Kennelly, and Karl Hankin. A special thanks to Equinox Fitness Clubs of NYC for their support.

This book would not have been possible without the help of Deb Killmon, Annette Lang, and James Villepigue.

Finally, I'd like to thank the Buddy Evans. If someone could harvest Buddy's energy, they could light up a major city. But the most remarkable thing about Buddy (other than the fact that he could stand on the ball on his first try) is that he overcame a life-threatening illness. Buddy is a solid surfer, a wonderful role model, and a shining example of how important the power of strong, positive energy can be in overcoming and recapturing a healthy life.

May we all surf long and strong!

Paul Frediani

CONTENTS

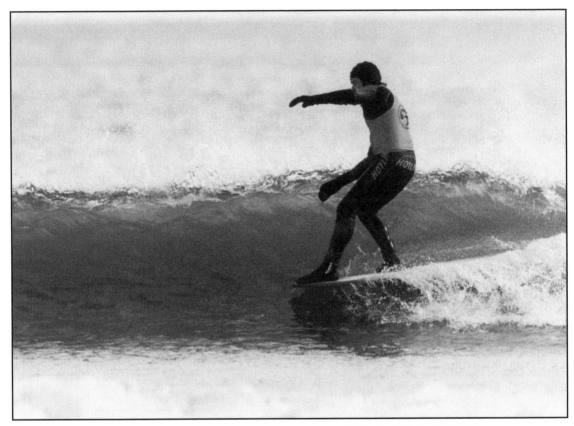

THE LEGENDARY PETER PAN RIDES THE NOSE. PHOTO BY JOE McGOVERN.

FOREWORD

BY JIM LUCAS

S urfing is the only life, the only life for me . . . " continues to be my mantra from that Beach Boys hit from the early '60s. With over 35 years surfing in search of that Holy Grail, the Perfect Wave, I have had the fortune to experience vast cultures and phenomenal waves the world over. Approaching my half-century birthdate, I still have the same fervor and enthusiasm as when I first stood up on a surfboard across a moving wall of water at Inside Pleasure Point, Santa Cruz, in 1964.

Whether you are a teenager or approaching the "autumn" of your life, physical shape and conditioning is an integral part of enjoying the surfing experience. What the author of this book provides is an all encompassing perspective of what all surfers, from grommet to kahuna, novice to expert, should do to keep surfing enjoyable.

The book covers conditioning, flexibility, workouts for both sexes, creating a workout schedule, and the prevention and treatment of common surf injuries.

Flexibility and conditioning is most obvious in a competitive environment. But it doesn't stop there. Whether you're off in darkest Baja, hundreds of miles away from the nearest doctor, or at your local break a stone's throw from the finest hospital, good conditioning and flexibility can prevent an unnecessary emergency trip or casualty.

Picture this: You're at your local break and a set wave is approaching. You're out of position, slightly inside. The local demon is dropping in, headed right for you. How will you fare if you have arms of spaghetti? Or what will your teenager think after a session go-out if afterwards you have to spend the rest of the day laid out on the couch? Exaggerated instances? Maybe yes. Maybe no.

What this book will provide is how to avoid those situations. This book will put you on a workout regimen that will keep you hitting the surf for years to come while your peers will be barely able to push the shuffleboard paddle.

Perhaps Mike Love and Brian Wilson may not have had the insight to fully grasp those words of wisdom—surfing truly is the only life. Read this book to make the most of yours.

Cowabunga forever,

Jim Lucas
Santa Cruz, California

ABOUT JIM LUCAS

Jim Lucas truly is a representative of California's surfing culture. During the late '60s and early '70s, Jim became one of the Soul Patrol—a group of Santa Cruz surfers who trekked up and down the North Coast in search of empty perfect waves. In the early '80s Jim became one of the first members of Surfrider Foundation, an organization to help save the nearshore environment. Also during the early '80s, he became a charter member, and eventually president, of the Big Stick Surfing Association, a longboard club dedicated to friendship and camaraderie in the spirit of the late Duke Kahanamoku. Jim's competitive surfing exploits have had him placing in numerous longboard contests throughout California, Hawaii, Japan, France, and Costa Rica. He is Team Captain of the Greg Noll/Da Bull Clothing Surf Team. He also founded and continues to direct the Surf-O-Rama, a longboard contest in which participants have to ride boards manufactured prior to 1969. Established in 1989, the Surf-O-Rama has raised over $50,000 to date for charity.

Jim was also a highly ranked high school and college wrestler in California, making two US Junior teams. Jim currently wrestles in the Masters division and placed 2nd at the AAU Masters Grand Nationals in 1997, 3rd in 1998 and 1999 and 2nd in the 2000 USA Wrestling Veterans National Championships. Jim has also placed multiple times in the Veterans World Championships. He coaches wrestling at Harbor High School in Santa Cruz.

Jim has written numerous articles for *Surfer Magazine*, *Longboard Magazine*, *Longboarder Magazine*, and *Classic Longboard Collector*. Jim also writes for *Wrestling Institute Newsmagazine* on the Masters/Veterans wrestling scene.

INTRODUCTION

*Surfing involves the entire body and mind. It's an immediate sport.
Once you commit to a wave, you're immediately involved in a moving, constantly changing playing field. You need arm and upper
body strength for paddling out, leg strength for balancing on the
board, and excellent lung capacity.*

—Tom McBride, who started board surfing in 1956 at Malibu, California.
An active board surfer for 20 years, at 61 Tom is in good shape and still
body surfs (sans board) in and around Carpinteria, California.

I can still remember my first days of surfing: It's 1964, and I'm sitting in
the back seat of a '58 Chevy convertible with my best friend Richie.
The surfboards are slid over the top of the passenger's seat, Richie's
blonde bombshell sister is driving, music is blasting, and Richie and I
are laughing with nervous expectation of a day of waves. Surfing the
icy waters of the San Francisco coastline, with just the top of a long-
sleeve wet suit, we were so cold our knees turned blue. But it didn't
matter because we were surfing—it was better than anything I had
experienced in my young life. We were on top of the world!

Now that I'm in my 40s, those feelings of excitation still return to
me whenever I smell surf wax, check out the local surf shop, or read
the latest surf magazines. It blows my mind to watch the hot young
kids today, just as it blew my mind back in the '60s watching the
greats then. Different styles, same passion.

It's been said, "Once a surfer, always a surfer." I believe it. Once
you're able to stand up on a wave, harness its energy, and ride it to

shore, you're hooked. It's almost impossible to explain to a non-surfer the sense of liberty and freedom you get from standing on a plank of fiberglass, screaming down a wall of emerald green water, roaring white water on your heels, wind-feathered salt water spraying you down. Some dedicate their lives to such passions.

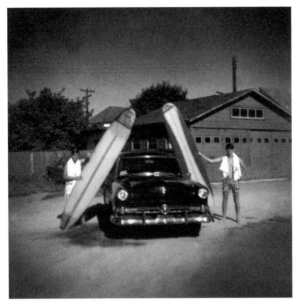

When I was a kid my dream was to spend my life driving up and down the San Mateo coastline looking for waves. Unfortunately, life got in the way, and now I have other passions. But surfing, like your first girlfriend, you never forget. I still surf, and some days it's not about riding the waves but just paddling out and enjoying the environment, a form of peace and meditation, sitting outside and rolling with the swells.

THE AUTHOR AND HIS BROTHER ENRICO, SANTA CRUZ, 1964.

My son Paolo learned to surf when he spent summers with me in Santa Monica. It has been a passion we've shared. Even when he was a teenager we had something to talk about, a common language (and those of you who have teenagers know that's not always easy to achieve). He also had a dream to be able to live and surf at the beach, and, unlike me, he has fulfilled his dream. He now lives right across the street from Ocean Beach. I know that if he has children, he'll teach them to surf. My wish is that from one generation to another we learn to love and respect the ocean.

I hope that by writing this book I can reach surfers of all generations. If you're a young thrasher looking to increase your conditioning, these workouts will help keep you healthy for a lifetime. If you're an older surfer, who's feeling the aches and pains in your joints and lower back, these workouts and stretches will get you back in the water, and you'll surf longer and stronger.

Those of us who surf know it's much more than a sport. Because when we place our feet on sand once again and turn our backs to the Big Blue, we know we'll be back, and she'll be waiting for us: to welcome, embrace, thrill, humiliate and entertain. A smile grows on our face as we walk away, making footprints in the sand. Because deeply buried in our gray matter, we acknowledge we belong there, and going back is like going home.

THE IMPORTANCE OF CONDITIONING

Strength, flexibility, cardiovascular, and balance (or "neural-muscular") conditioning are essential for surfing. You need strength, endurance, and cardio capacity to paddle out through the breakers, flexibility to surf longer and stronger, and balance to surf fluidly.

Here's a scenario that most surfers have experienced: You've just mastered an awesome wave, have a great ride to shore, and you turn around to paddle back out, working hard to get beyond the impact zone. You get yourself back in the line-up, but just as you take a break to catch your breath, someone yells "outside," and everyone is scrambling to get positioned for the incoming set.

You turn and paddle like mad, your lungs burning, your arms feeling like wet noodles, and you just make it in time to position yourself

3

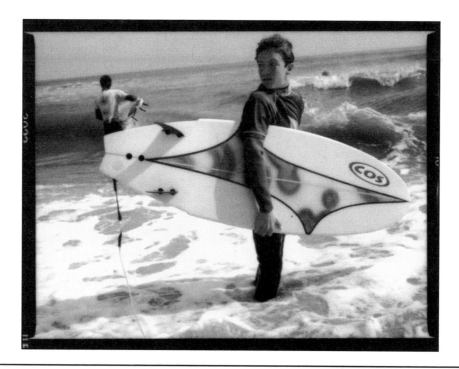

for the last wave of the set. It's a beauty! Your arms have just enough strength left for you to catch the wave. You pop up—and then literally just fall off. Being physically depleted, your balance is shot (your neural-muscular system is burnt). Now you have to deal with being bounced and bent like a pretzel, all the while holding your breath under water.

"Yeah, man, surfing sure is fun," you might be thinking, while your lungs are bursting and you're looking for the surface. Or maybe you're thinking, "Gee, maybe if I wasn't so exhausted, I wouldn't have collapsed on that wave. Maybe I should get myself in better condition."

Well, here's how.

4

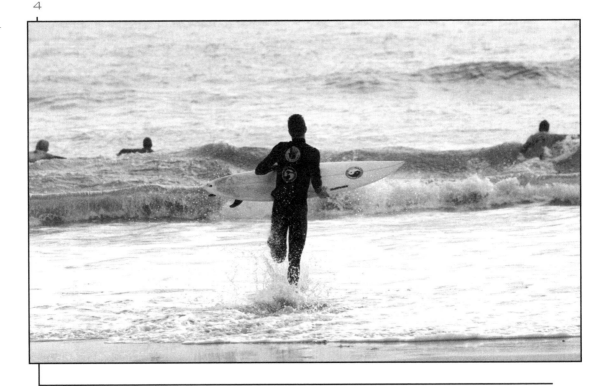

2

FLEX TIME

After more than 20 years' surfing, there has been no greater force in extending the quality and performance of my surfing than to have incorporated a stretching and yoga routine as part of my daily life.

—Jim Miller, 30-year-old surf instructor/ocean lifeguard, Manhattan Beach, CA, www.puresurfingexperience.com

W e all know how important flexibility and stretching is, not only for surfing but also for maintaining a healthy and active lifestyle in which we can move freely and painlessly with a full range of motion. Unfortunately, stretching is a lot like eating broccoli—we know its good for us, but man, it's hard to swallow. If you're committed to keeping surfing as an important part of your life, you've got to commit yourself to flexibility training.

As we grow older, our muscles and joints naturally tighten up. Though we think that surfing gets us in shape, the fact is that surfing, because of its repetitive paddling motion, develops muscle imbalances. If you choose to ignore the symptoms or lack awareness of these imbalances, it will lead to injury. You can stop surfing for a while to recover, and perhaps see a doctor or chiropractor for help with your problems, but once you start surfing again, the same imbalances will appear, and the same injury will return.

Constant paddling creates tight shoulder and chest muscles, developing that forward-slumping shoulder posture known as "upper cross syndrome." This poor posture can develop an unstable shoulder girdle, which in turn can develop into impingement in your rotator cuff, causing inflammation and pain when you paddle. Paddling is also the reason so many surfers have bad backs and sore necks. Lying on your board with your chest high and your back hyperextended creates pressure in your lower back and tension in your neck.

Tight hips (hip flexor muscles) also make your back tight. Inflexible hamstrings and quadriceps can keep you from doing a quick and smooth pop-up, and you definitely won't be able to get into a squatting cheater five position and get up gracefully. Having tight leg muscles can also create bad tracking of the knee (patella), causing pain and discomfort. And all this doesn't even address the kind of contortions your body goes through in a wipe-out.

Isn't it worth a few minutes a day to avoid injuries that can become chronic and deprive you of going in the water? In the later portion of this chapter you can assess your flexibility. Some of the most effective and efficient stretches surfers can do are yoga sun salutations. Not only do they stretch you in a sports-specific matter (flexion, extension, and rotation of your spine, hips, and legs), they also give you a superb warm-up and engage your neural-muscular system (for balance).

The following basic sun salutations are straightforward and easy to follow so you can begin to develop better body awareness and understanding of your flexibility needs. Included are simple but practical stretches surfers can incorporate into their daily living activities. Remember to consult your doctor before trying these stretches. Stretching is not a competition—do it at your own level. Enjoy each stretch; stretching is good. Breathe, relax, and smile. After all, how many people are lucky enough to surf!

Following the Pre-Surf Salutations, which you do before you paddle out, are a series of Everyday Stretches you can do before you even get out of bed in the morning—as well as before or after the conditioning exercises described in the following chapters. The stretches are designed to hit every major muscle group.

SURF THERAPY YOGA

BY CHARLES S. DEFAY

No active or enthusiastic surfer on the planet does *not* want to surf as long as possible. The rigors of a surfing lifestyle—stamina, flexibility, breath control, body weight, balance, and even the wellness of the mind—are so *critical* to a surfer's longevity and the quality of his performance.

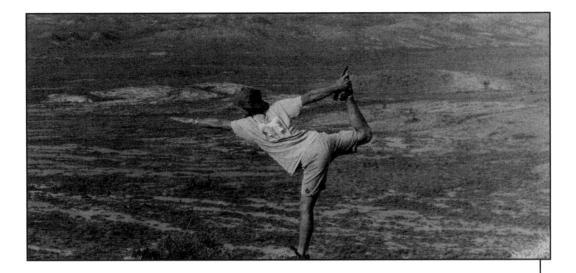

The practice of Hatha Yoga (based on the balance of opposites such as the sun and the moon) can greatly improve a surfer's endurance and physical strength. Hatha Yoga is the ultimate all-around physical and mental preparation for the act of surfing, or any other physical activity for that matter.

The ancient Rishis (wise sages from pre-biblical times) designed the Asanas (the physical postures) to optimize the health of the body temple for the arduous battles of life and for the great length of time it takes to advance our consciousness and spirit. Optimum health in the body, mind and soul is the purpose of Hatha Yoga. Hatha Yoga is a highly disciplined practice that transforms and purifies the body temple, making it fit as a tool for self-discovery.

On a much deeper level, the practice of yoga is eight-fold. Listed below are eight steps:

1. **Yama**—moral conduct/self-control (avoiding all things that make us unhappy)
2. **Niyama**—adherence (association with positive qualities such as right action, right speech, or a healthy association with people)
3. **Asanas**—physical postures
4. **Pranayama**—breath control (life force control)
5. **Pratyahara**—internalization
6. **Dharana**—concentration

7. **Dhyana**—meditation

8. **Samadhi**—supreme consciousness/god consciousness

The eight-fold path is inclusive, aligning the body, mind and emotion with the true essence of our souls. One cannot meditate nor do Asanas without addressing all of their personal issues (i.e., emotional blocks). Yoga is a lifelong therapy in itself. One cannot act immorally (i.e., cheat, lie, or steal) and be able to meditate. The Tishis' design of the Asanas makes the body temple strong enough and healthy enough to sit still and meditate for long periods of time (with disciplined practice). All of the steps of the eight-fold path are applicable at all times and each step is interdependent. A surfer will find it harder to enjoy surfing if they are acting immoral in the surf or in their lives. However, respect, generosity, and humility all add to the possibility of a greater connection with their fellow man, nature, and the forces of the spirit.

In a yoga posture, every ligament, tissue, tendon, muscle, bone, and complex system in the body opens. With an awareness of the internal current, focus, concentration and physical effort (honoring physical limitations) heightens with conscious practice. Very importantly, oxygenation and cleansing of every cell occurs with practice. Aging, disease, and inflexibility are generally due to stagnation (lack of Prana life force) in those body parts.

There is a saying in yoga: you are only as old as your spine is flexible. Yoga progress is based on gentle persistence over time. Each asana has a particular scientific physical emphasis, whether it is organ cleansing and stimulation, spinal alignment, or balancing of the blood pressure. The benefits are endless! The practice of Asanas is 99 percent practice and one percent theory (for all eight steps). Surfing is the same, 99 percent experiential and one percent theory. My ongoing practice of Asanas and mediation (Sadhana) continue to strengthen my physical and spiritual energy.

YOGA PRE-SURF SALUTIONS

The American Academy of Orthopedic Surgeons recommends warming up and stretching before physical activities to prevent injuries. The following stretches are a perfect blend of stretching and warm-up with the added benefit of breathing exercises.

Charles S. DeFay is currently a senior Synergy Yoga teacher at the Yoga Room in Encinitas, California and studies with Peri Ness, founder and master teacher of Synergy Yoga and the newly formed Synergy Yoga University. Charles has practiced Hatha Yoga for over 25 years and has been teaching for five years. He has been an active surfer for 37 years in California, Hawaii, and Latin America. He currently resides in Point Arena, California where he teaches Synergy Yoga at Surf Therapy Yoga, his own business. He received a B.S. degree in geology from San Diego State University in 1976. He was a beach lifeguard in Coronado, in the city of San Diego, from 1969 to 1972, and the captain of the lifeguard service from 1973 to 1977. He has practiced transformational bodywork therapy from 1990 to the present. Charles is a member of self-realization fellowship, founded by Parmahansa Yogananda, which emphasizes Kriya Yoga; an advanced meditation technique designed to speed up the spiritual progress.

To learn more about Synergy Yoga or to purchase a video, go to www.synergy-yoga.com.

The word yoga means union and it is a practice that will integrate your body, mind and breath. A consistent practice will rejuvenate your mind, reduce stress, create mental clarity and provide relaxation. Yoga will help heal and avoid repetitive stress injuries. It will ground you to the earth, improving your balance through your relationship with gravity. Steady practice will increase your core strength and stability. This is crucial in maintaining a healthy back. Yoga will encourage the release of unhealthy muscle tension and help correct poor movement patterns that can create bad posture (such as the upper cross syndrome in surfers). Bad posture can create greater wear and tear on the joints and diminishes athletic performance.

Yoga will also cultivate and promote deep breathing, an indispensable necessity for surfers. Deep and proper breathing will keep your mind clear and your body relaxed. It will keep you loose in tight situations and can save your life. Proper breathing improves the delivery of oxygen and nutrients to muscles and tissues, which is essential for optimum health. The key element to focus on while doing these salutations is your breathing! Holding your breath will make you more tense.

PRE-SURF SALUTATIONS

The following pre-surf stretches are yoga poses that focus on flexion, extension and rotation. Preparing your body for the movement required in surfing. Begin slowly as you learn each pose.

With each pose, you should feel the gradual lengthening of your muscles and the release of tension. Breathe deeply through your nose. Draw your breath down to your lower abdominals and lower back, expanding your lower ribcage. Allow your diaphragm to drop lower in the abdominal cavity, providing more room for your lungs to reach full capacity. Exhale through the back of your throat and out your mouth and nose. Remember to keep your facial muscles relaxed and your shoulders down and away from your ears.

Stretching may be a little uncomfortable but should never be painful. None of these poses should cause pain. If they do, back off, and do them in the range of motion that is pain-free. Perform these stretches consecutively so that one pose leads to the next. You can hold these stretches for an extended period of time up to 20 seconds, or they can be held for five inhales and five exhales each.

As you become familiar with the series of salutations, increase the rhythm and decrease the amount of time you hold each pose. This will provide you with an excellent preparation for your surf session. Doing the pre-surf salutation at a quicker pace will not only warm you up and stretch you out, it will also get your nervous system prepared to work toward the speed of movement that is required in actual surfing.

Start slowly, holding each pose for 10 to 20 seconds. After you have familiarized yourself with the stretches and routine, cycle through the poses with minimum pause at each stretch. By moving through the routine in this fashion 5 to 10 times, you get not only a great stretch, but also an excellent warm-up.

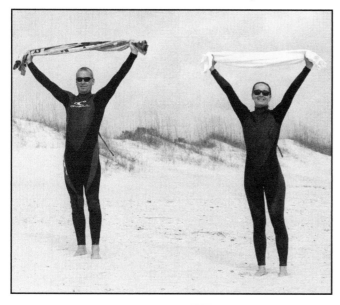

TOWEL STRETCH

Stand straight with your feet together while holding either end of a towel in your hands. Keeping the towel taut, bring it up and over your head and down behind your back. Repeat the motion holding the towel vertically making sure to keep your abs and buttocks tight, stretching your chest and shoulders.

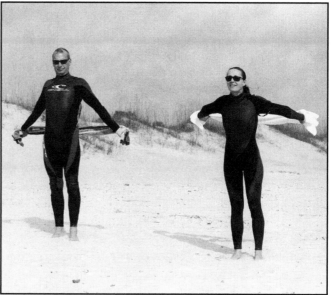

SUN SALUTATION

Stand straight with your feet together, head facing forward. Put your palms together in a prayer position at your chest, then raise them directly over your head, stretching your arms as high as you can and bend backwards. Go slowly and only in your own comfort zone.

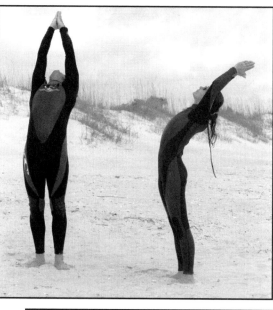

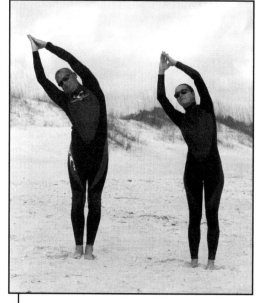

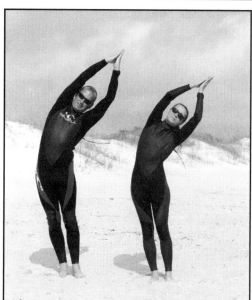

SIDE BENDS

From the sun salutation position, bend to your right side, hold the pose, then bend to your left side and hold the pose. Return your arms directly over your head. Lift your top ribs as high as you can, stretching your intercostales (chest) and giving your lungs room to expand. Side bends will also stretch your waist and latissimus dorsi (the big paddling muscles on the sides of your back). By crossing your feet, you can also stretch the outside of your hips.

FORWARD BEND

Keeping your knees slightly bent, bend your torso forward, keeping your arms outstretched in front of your head. If you have good flexibility, straighten your knees. Let your breath fill your lower back. As you exhale, tighten your stomach. This will allow you to go a little deeper into the stretch. This stretches your lower back, glutes, and hamstrings.

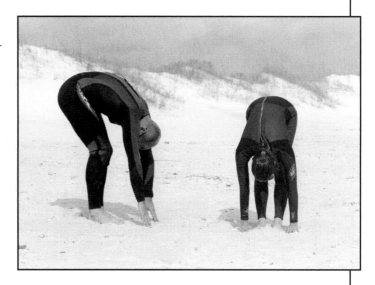

RUNNER'S POSE

Extend your right foot behind you and place your hands on the ground. As you exhale, press your hips to the ground. Bring your feet back together, lean into a forward bend, and then drop your left foot behind you and repeat the stretch. For a deeper stretch, bring your elbows to the ground. This is an excellent stretch for your groin, hip flexor, and hamstring.

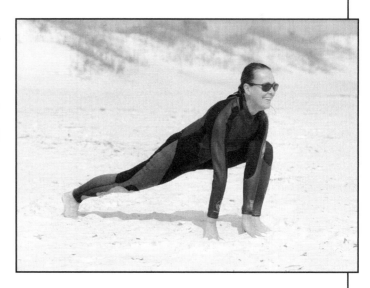

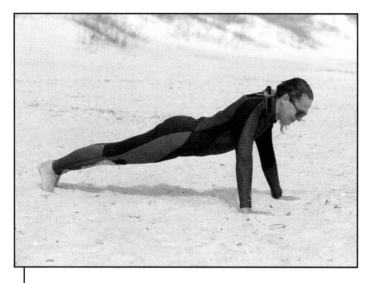

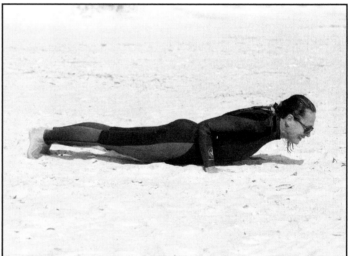

PLANK POSE

Place both hands directly under your shoulders, and extend both legs out behind you. Lower your chest to the ground. Avoid dipping your lower back. If your back is swaying, place your knees on the ground as you perform this exercise. This is an overall body-strengthening pose.

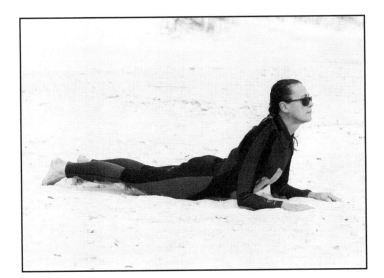

COBRA POSE

From the Plank Pose position, lower your hips to the ground. Engage your back muscles to lift your chest, then straighten your arms and push your chest out between your arms. Keep your shoulder down and back. If this position puts too much stress on your lower back, keep your elbows bent and on the ground. This pose stretches your abdominals and chest, and strengthens your back.

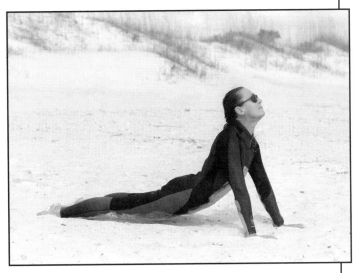

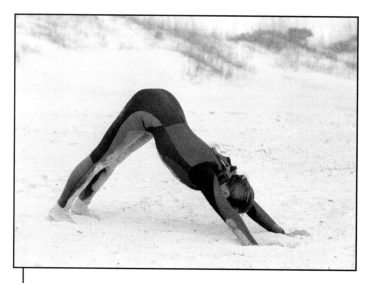

DOWNWARD-FACING DOG

From the Cobra Pose, lift your hips up and back, pressing your heels into the ground and squeezing your shoulder blades together. This is an excellent resting pose and it stretches the back of the legs, shoulders and chest.

WARRIOR POSE—BEGINNER

From the Downward-Facing Dog Pose, step forward with your right foot. Raise your head and torso and stretch your right arm over your right knee and your left arm over your left leg. Your left foot should be at a 90-degree angle to your right heel. Press your left hip forward. As you exhale, bend your right knee to increase your stretch. Keep your left leg strong, supportive and active. Bring your feet back together, lower your body into the Plank Pose, and then return to the Downward-Facing Dog position. Repeat this pose with your right leg back. This is an overall leg and core-strengthening pose, which stretches your inner thighs, hip flexors and groin.

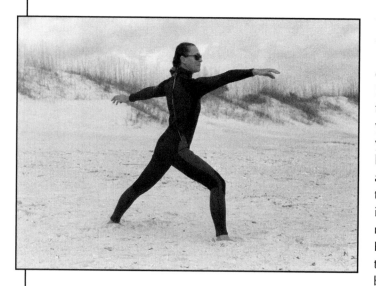

WARRIOR POSE—
INTERMEDIATE

From the beginning Warrior Pose with your right leg forward, turn your hips, torso, head and arms to the right. Place your hands in front of your chest in a prayer position. Place your left elbow on the outside of your right thigh. Concentrate on maintaining your balance and the rotation of the torso. This pose strengthens the legs and butt and stretches the groin, shoulders, and hip flexors.

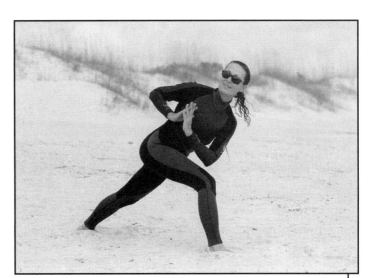

TRIANGLE POSE

From the Warrior Pose, rotate your torso to the right, keeping your arm and legs strong and lengthening your spine. Let your legs (not your left hand) support you. Look up to your right hand and keep your ribs elevated.

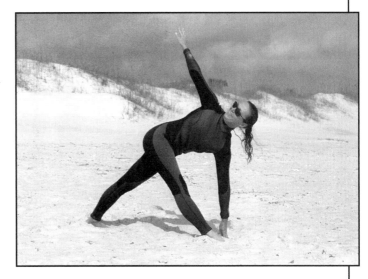

EVERYDAY STRETCHES

The following everyday stretches are simple and easy to do. I recommend doing them everyday before getting out of bed. Your back will love you for it! These stretches will promote a healthy and supple spine. To keep your shoulders healthy, do the stretches on page 119 and 120. If you do these stretches regularly, it will help counterbalance the muscles used in paddling, and help avoid tight shoulder muscles. It's a good idea to do the shoulder stretches before and after each surf session. Hold each stretch for 20 to 30 seconds, breathe deeply, and increase the stretch slightly as you exhale.

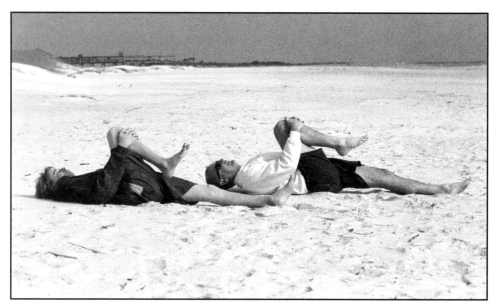

Lie on your back on the ground (or on your bed), with your legs fully extended. Bring one knee to your chest, holding it with your hands. Repeat with the opposite knee. Then, bring both knees to your chest simultaneously. This is an excellent stretch for your back.

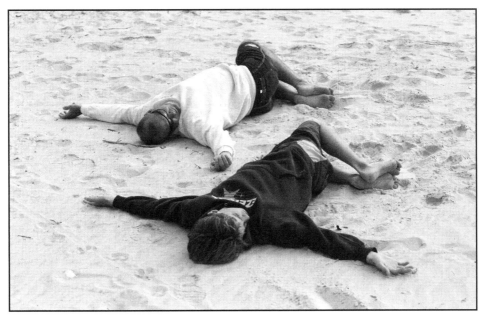

From that position, roll both knees to your left side, keeping both your shoulders on the floor. Stretch your right arm out to the side. Repeat on the opposite side. Spinal rotation is essential for surfing.

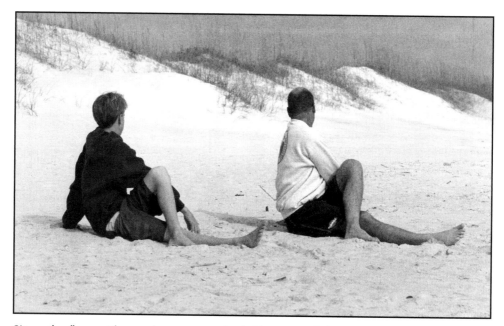

Sit on the floor with your legs outstretched. Place your left foot on the far side of your right knee, and twist your torso to face left. Keep your back straight and abdominals tight. Use your left hand for stability, as shown. Repeat on the opposite side.

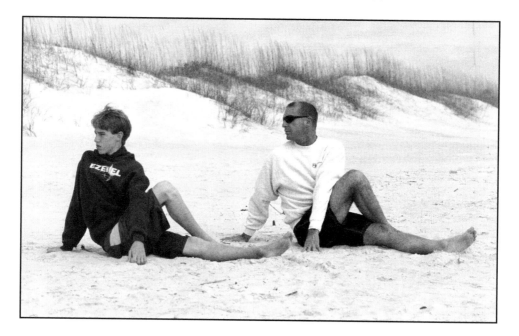

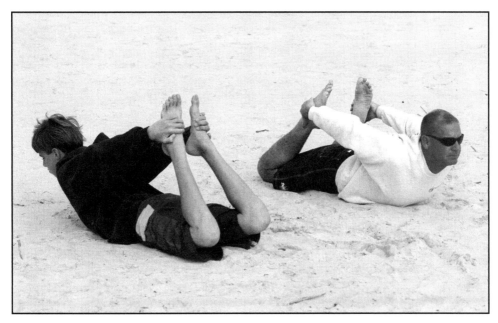

Advanced: Lie on your stomach on the floor with your legs outstretched. Bending your knees, grab both feet and lift your head off the ground. Squeeze your shoulders back, engage your buttocks and rock back and forth. For a more basic move, start by holding one foot. This stretch will work your hips, quads, chest and back.

FLEXIBILITY ASSESSMENT

Annette Lang, program director for Esquerre Fitness Group International, and a Reebok University Master Trainer, recommends some simple assessments for flexibility and mobility. Flexibility (stretching) is needed if you have a tight muscle that may be limiting the amount of movement you can do, whether surfing or not. For example, if your chest and shoulder muscles are tight, it could limit the amount of arm movement you have to bring you out to the surf. Tight hamstrings and lower back muscles can limit the amount of time you can hold your position on the surfboard before getting tired.

Mobility on the other hand, is a general limitation of the whole area. You may just feel like you are stiff and slow during your movements, or you can't get into certain positions smoothly. For example, if you always turn in one direction while surfing, you may feel "tight" when trying to move in the other direction. When you need mobility, you might feel more like you "just can't get there" than tightness in one particular muscle.

The stretches and mobility exercises that follow will address both issues: stretching for the individual muscles, and mobility exercises to get your body moving more freely and easily. For more information on mobility and flexibility, go to www.esquerrefitnessgroup.com.

Flexibility Assessment—To assess your own flexibility, try one of these seven poses. Difficulty with any of them indicates a lack of flexibility in the muscles or in the mobility of the joint.

HAMSTRINGS

Lie on your back on the floor. Lift one leg straight up so that it is perpendicular to your body, i.e., at a right angle to your body. Keep the opposite leg straight. If you have

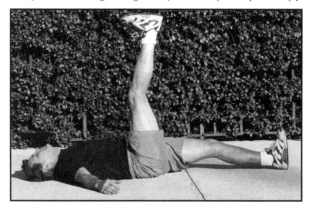

difficulty raising either leg up to a right angle, you probably have tight hamstrings and will benefit from the first Everyday Stretch and several of the Pre-Surf Salutations, especially the Downward-Facing Dog. Also try the Swiss Ball Hamstring Stretch.

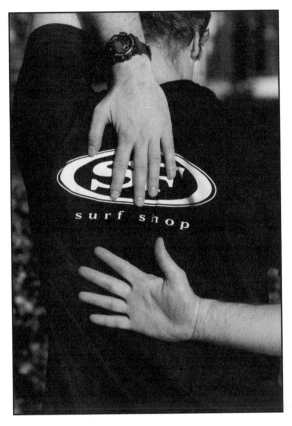

SHOULDERS

Place one hand, palm facing outward, on your back and reach the other hand up and behind your head, as shown. Repeat with the opposite arms. (The second photo shows how the stretch looks if your muscles around the shoulders are tight.) If you have difficulty with this stretch or lack shoulder mobility, see the Wahine chapter and yoga workout.

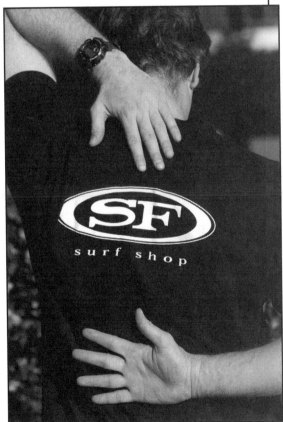

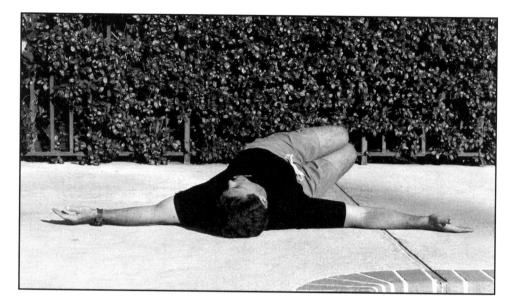

SPINE AND HIPS

Lie on your back on the floor and stretch your arms out so that they're perpendicular to your body. Keeping your head on the floor, raise your legs so that they form a 90 degree angle at the hips and a 90 degree angle at the knees. Let your knees fall to one side of your body. Can you keep both your shoulders on the ground? Repeat, letting your knees fall to the opposite side. If you have trouble keeping your shoulders on the ground, in essence moving your hips and shoulders in opposite directions, you could benefit from a spinal rotation exercise. Also try the Swiss Ball Hip and Lower Back Stretch, and the Swiss Ball Spinal Rotation.

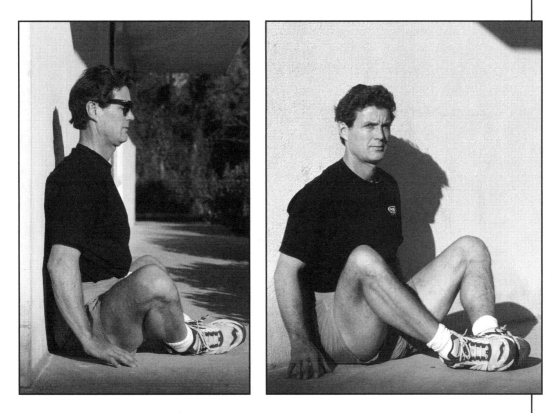

INNER THIGHS AND HIPS

Sit with your back against the wall. Making sure your lower back is touching the wall, bring your feet as far in toward your groin as they can go. Your knees should be half way to the ground (i.e., at a 45 degree angle). If you have difficulty with this pose, your inner thigh muscles might be tight, and you could benefit from this stretch as well as side lunges. (The second photo shows the tight stretch.) Also try the Swiss Ball Hip and Groin Stretch.

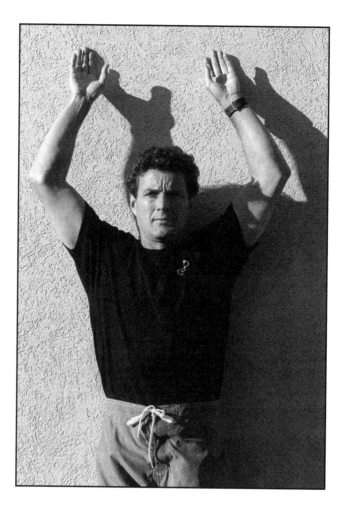

BACK

Stand against a wall so that your feet are about a foot from the wall and your butt is touching the wall. Keeping your lower back against the wall, raise your arms up over your head. Can you keep your arms straight and in contact with the wall without arching your back? If you have tightness, a way to increase mobility and flexibility is to sit against the wall in this position, with your elbows at shoulder height, and slowly "walk" your arms up and down the wall. Also try the Lower Back Stretch and the Waist Stretch to target the lats.

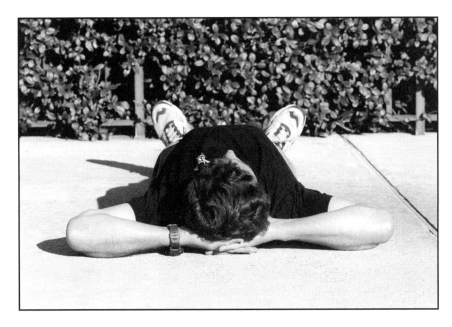

CHEST

Lie on your back with your hands behind your head. Do your elbows touch the ground? If not, you could benefit from some chest stretches. (The second photo shows the tightness of the chest.) Also try the Swiss Ball Chest Stretch.

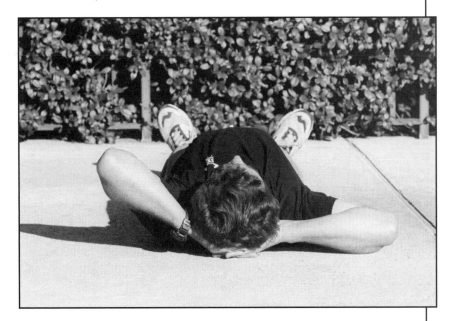

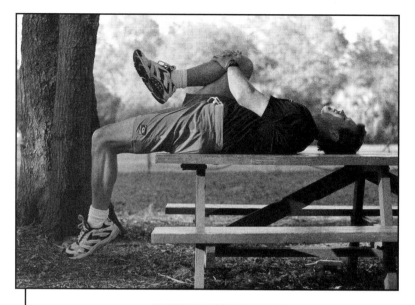

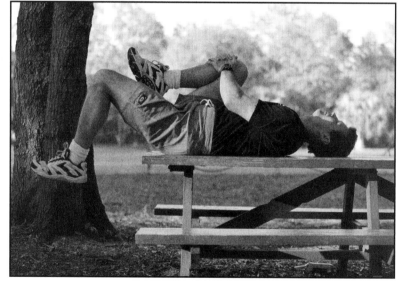

QUAD AND HIP FLEXORS

Lie with your hips on the edge of a bench. Grab one knee and pull it up toward your chest, while keeping the other leg bent at 90 degrees off the bench. Repeat with the other leg. Lunge stretches can help prevent difficulty with this move. (The second photo shows tightness.) Also try the Swiss Ball Quad Stretch.

3

THE SURF FLEX
WORKOUT

*Before surfing I always jump up and down in the sand
for about three to four minutes. It helps to stretch out my legs,
back, and feet and really gets my breathing going. Doing a few
windmills with the arms never hurts either.*

—Corky Carroll, three-time International Professional Surfing Champion,
five-time United States Surfing Champion,
and former No. 1 Surfer in the World

T he Surf Flex Workout uses a Swiss Ball, one of the most versatile pieces of equipment used today (i.e., "stability balls", "Fit-balls", Physioballs", etc.). Since the 1960s, Swiss Balls have been used with great success in the rehabilitative setting. Since 1980, due to their effectiveness in developing balance and core strength, they have become the new craze in the world of fitness and athletic conditioning. This performance enhancement tool is available at most gyms and sporting good stores. Be sure to choose a ball that's the right size for your physique. Ideally, when you sit on the ball a 90-degree angle should form at your hips and knees. However, it's good practice to train on balls of all sizes for greater strength and flexibility (smaller for strength, larger for flexibility).

This unique form of training will challenge your strength, endurance and balance by utilizing your neuromuscular system (i.e., your brain tells your muscles how to move and how to keep your balance).

Surf Flex will help you develop strength of "core" (abdominal, back, hip) muscles that are vital for surfing performance. The Swiss Ball routines are the ultimate way to strengthen your stabilizing muscles, which are found at the body's major joints, namely around the spine, hips and shoulders. Strong stabilizing muscles allow your body to move more powerfully, fluidly and with less chance of injury.

First, let's review some "core" concepts to help you understand why Surf Flex training is so beneficial. What is the core of your body? Like the core of an apple, your core is your foundation or support system for your entire body. It is your spine, plus your pelvic and shoulder girdles, and the muscles that act on these bony structures (i.e., back and hip muscles). However, generally the core refers to the abdominal and lower back muscles.

Why should you train your core? Well, your core muscles stabilize your spine and connect your upper and lower extremities, or more simply, your hips and shoulders. As a result, optimum functioning of your limbs is dependent on your core strength and stability (i.e., "proximal stability" around your spine, shoulders and pelvis promotes "distal mobility" of your arms and legs). Your core is also your center of power, and is essential for the efficient transfer of force and the development of efficient movement. Many researchers believe it is where all movement begins.

Furthermore, your core is where your center of gravity is located, and therefore, plays an essential role in maintaining balance and equilibrium. It is also involved in respiration at rest and during exercise, and your abdominal muscles provide intra-abdominal pressure to support your spine and decrease the incidence of lower back injuries. Finally, the healthier your core the better your posture, which will help you look and feel better. In essence, a strong and stable core is key for optimum performance in daily living, exercise, and sports, especially surfing!

Okay, so we know that Surf Flex will improve your core strength and stability, but there's more good news, it will also improve your function! The Surf Flex Workout is functional training, or movement training that will help you be better prepared for the demands of daily life, work activities, and sports performance. Functional exercises on the ball can simulate surfing movements - from paddling out, popping up, or rotating around the pipe of a giant wave. Functional exercises also help counteract muscle imbalances in strength and/or flexibility, enhance coordination, and improve your balance and proprioception, or sense of where your body is in space.

This unique training system will excite your nervous system and challenge your body with movements that challenge your base of support in an unstable environment—just like surfing in the sea! Exercises on the Swiss Ball will force you to engage the muscles that stabilize your spine, shoulders, hips, knees, and ankles optimally. The Surf Flex Workout will encourage your body to work as a functional unit with a strong stable core, and will improve your surfing performance!

Now on to the fun stuff! However, before attempting any advanced moves, take the ab strength test below:

AB STRENGTH TEST

1. Lie on your back with your hands clasped behind your head and your legs flat on the floor in front of you. Can you do a full sit-up without lifting your legs or using forward momentum?

2. Lie on your back with your arms to the sides. Lift your legs out 90 degrees with your feet pointed toward the ceiling and your lower back pressed against the floor. Lower your legs slowly. Can you get lower your legs within a few inches of the floor without arching your back? Stop this test immediately if you notice your back arching.

3. How many bent-knee sit-ups can you do within one minute with your hands behind your head? Can you beat the average below?

AGE	SIT-UPS
20–29	40
30–39	30
40–45	25
46–55	20

If you answered "no" to these questions, you need to strengthen your abdominal muscles in a more conventional manner before attempting any advanced sit-ups on the Swiss Ball.

SECRETS TO SURF FLEX SUCCESS

A few key points to keep in mind…

1. Maintain a neutral spine. Always try to maintain the natural curves of your spine, from the base of your head to your tailbone.

2. Engage your abdominals. Think with your core, and be aware of pulling your navel to your spine without flattening the natural curve in your lower back. This will help strengthen your muscles, support your spine, decrease lower back injury, and improve your balance and posture. Do not let your lower back arch when performing exercises in a face down position.

3. Support. The longer the distance between support points (i.e., your hands/feet and the ball in a push-up) the harder the exercise. A wide leg position offers greater support; as your legs get closer to each other, you have less support and the exercise becomes harder. One leg-supported exercises are the hardest due to the additional support and balance demands.

4. Always exercise with a shirt. Sweaty bodies can easily slide off the ball, causing possible injury.

5. Challenge yourself and be consistent in your training. Try to maintain your balance longer, do a few more reps, and attempt to progress to the next level over time. The extra effort and continual practice will make a difference out on the surf!

> *Remember that training should be fun*
> and is ultimately a process
> for performance enhancement!

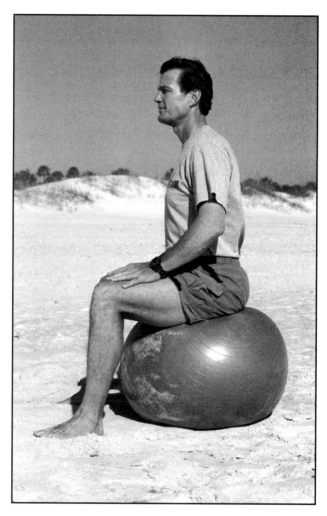

BODY ALIGNMENT

Always maintain a neutral spine position when doing any exercises on the Swiss Ball. Keep your chest high and your head aligned with your spine. Try using the Swiss Ball at your desk as a chair. It will improve your posture, strengthen your core, and even help eliminate carpal tunnel syndrome

THE WARM-UP

It is important to warm-up before your workout. The following exercises will help you connect with your core, increase your body temperature, and simultaneously improve your balance, strength and flexibility.

- Pelvic tilts: Front to back
                    Side to side
                    Circles (right/left)
                    Figure eights

*Sitting on the ball, warm up by tilting your pelvis in all directions.
*Perform 10 to 15 reps of each.

- Torso twists
- Torso diagonals

*Stand holding the ball and warm-up your entire body by twisting your torso side to side and on diagonal patterns (i.e., twist and look behind you; bring the ball to your right knee then over your left shoulder).
*Perform 10 to 15 reps of each.

Stretching: The following Swiss Ball flexibility exercises provide balance, coordination and strength training, in addition to preparing your body for further work. Hold each stretch for 15 to 20 seconds, relax and slowly breathe.

HOW TO SIZE A SWISS BALL

If your height is:	Choose this size:
up to 4'10" (145cm)	18" (45cm)
4'8" to 5'5" (140 - 165cm)	22" (55cm)
5'6" to 6'0" (165 - 185cm)	26" (65cm)
6'0" to 6'5" (185 - 195cm)	30" (75cm)
over 6'5" (195cm)	33" (85cm)

34

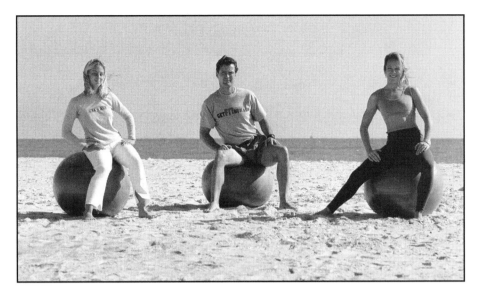

FIGURE EIGHTS

The key to performing all the Swiss Ball exercises correctly is to find and maintain a "neutral spine" position. In this position, your back is neither excessively rounded nor unnaturally swayed. To find your neutral spine position, sit erect on the ball and gently rock forward and back, then rock from side to side. As you come to a stop, tighten your abdominal muscles by pulling your navel to your spine. You should now be in neutral spine position. Doing Figure Eights is a wonderful way to massage your lower back.

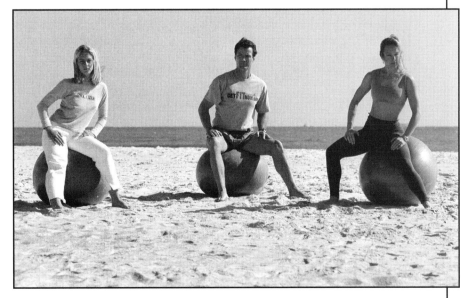

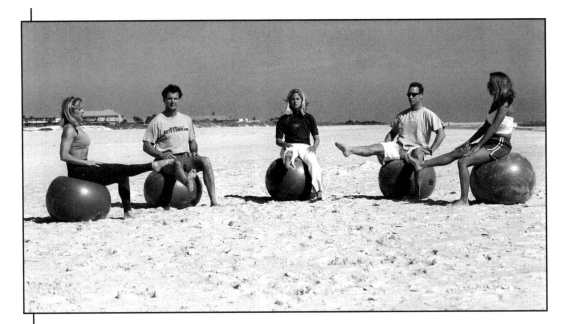

SITTING BALANCE

While sitting on the ball, try lifting one foot off the ground. It sounds a lot easier than it is. Sitting on your surfboard is a pretty easy task, if you've been surfing a while, but do you remember the first time you tried to sit on your board, being all cool in the line-up, and simply flipping off? Once you can balance on the ball while seated, you can proceed to a higher surfing progression.

Once you can comfortably balance on your knees, proceed to the following workout. This workout will challenge your strength, endurance, and balance. The more exhausted you become, the harder it will be to get back on the ball and maintain balance.

Pay special attention to your lower back—do not attempt the advanced versions until you have developed a strong lower back.

The first series of exercises are stretches. Hold each position for 10 to 20 seconds. In the case of strength exercises, like push-ups and lunges, do 5 to 10 reps just to get your blood pumping. (The full strength workout will follow.) If your back aches during any exercise, lessen the intensity. Always remind yourself to engage your abdominal muscles.

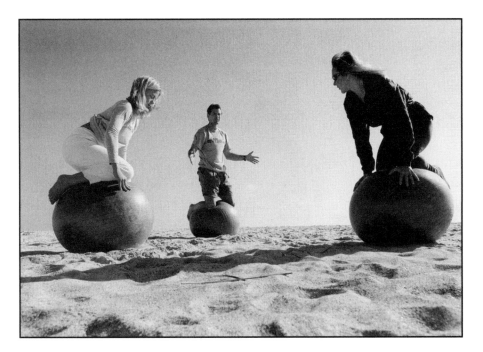

Another key position on the Swiss Ball is the kneeling position. First, place your feet shoulder-width apart behind the ball. Place one knee on top of the ball, then the other, and then place your hands on floor in front of you. Try to remove your hands from the floor and place them on the ball. This move alone usually takes many tries. Attempt it for only 5 minutes at a time.

Once you are comfortable with your hands and knees balanced on the ball, work toward taking your hands off the ball and raising your body up on your knees. Don't let frustration get in your way—everyone has his or her own timetable. It took me close to a month to feel comfortable on my knees, my brother took two weeks, and my son skipped the kneeling stage and stood up on his feet and balanced on the ball on his first try. Try to remember that finding or maintaining your balance is an ongoing process. As you

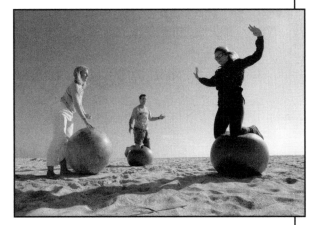

become skilled at maintaining your equilibrium, your point of balance will become wider and wider. Balance is the place where all movements begin and end.

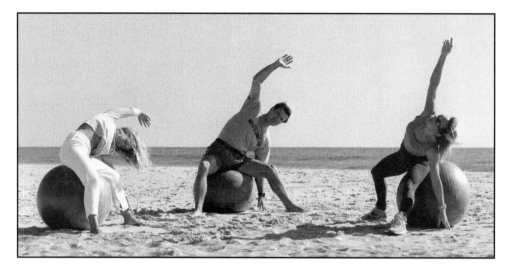

WAIST STRETCH

Sit on top of the ball with your feet wide apart, chest high, and shoulders back. With your arms outstretched, lean to one side and then the other. The waist stretch will help prepare your torso for the rotational movement that surfing demands. You can make this exercise a cardio workout by keeping your bottom hand on the ball while lifting your butt off of the ball. Reach your opposite hand over your head and alternate hands. Try one-minute sets for this excellent leg workout.

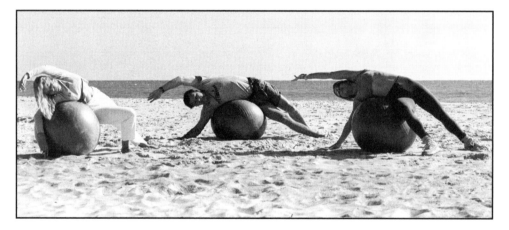

LOWER BACK STRETCH

With the side of your waist on the ball, split your legs for balance, put your lower hand on the ground, and reach the opposite hand over your head. This will not only stretch your back, hip, and waist, but will give a great and much needed stretch to the big paddling muscles (latissimus dorsi).

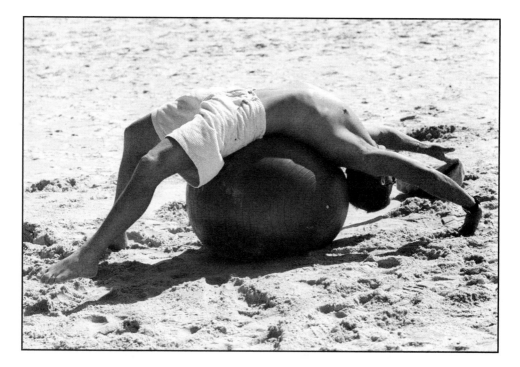

AB AND CHEST STRETCH

Start by sitting on the ball and rolling gently down to your lower back. Ease yourself back slowly. Increase your range by small increments. Never stretch if it's painful. Place your arms overhead to stretch your abs and out at 90 degrees to target your chest.

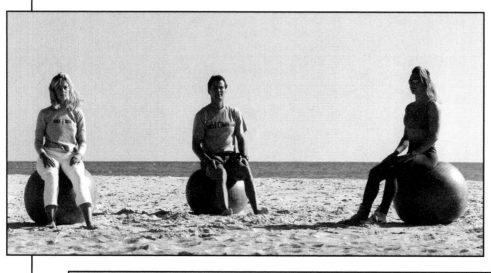

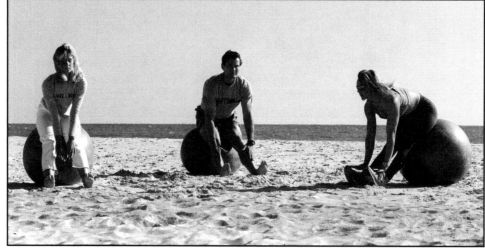

HAMSTRING STRETCH

Sit upright on ball with your knees bent. Straighten both your legs at the same time. Lift your toes to your shins and reach forward, bending at your waist. Do not hunch over! Keep your back flat. You will feel the stretch from your butt to your calves. Who doesn't have tight hamstrings? Stretching them well will help prevent a tight lower back.

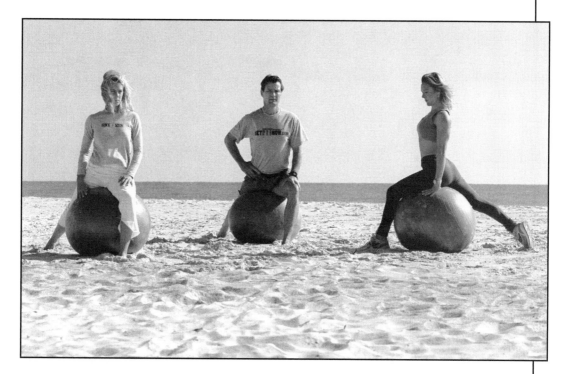

HIP AND GROIN STRETCH

Straddle the ball with one leg forward and one leg back. As you roll and press your back hip forward, you will stretch the groin and hip of your rear leg. If you press and roll back, you will stretch the back of your front leg. Flexible and strong hips generate powerful and snappy turns.

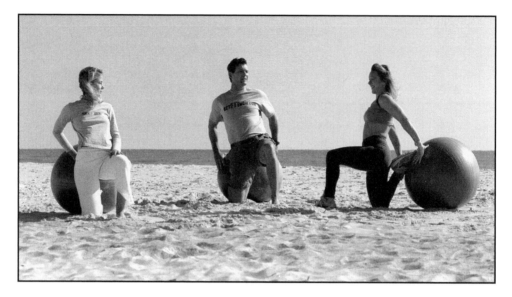

QUAD STRETCH

Place the top of your rear foot on the ball and place the other foot flat on the ground, with the knee bent at 90 degrees. As you lean back you will stretch the front of your hip and thigh. These muscles get tight easily—keeping them flexible will keep you in the water.

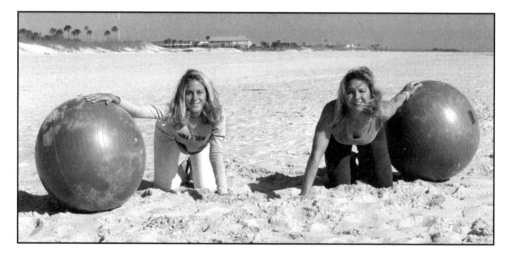

CHEST STRETCH

Kneel next to the ball and place one hand on top it. Press your chest down. Do this at a variety of angles to stretch different areas of your chest. Chest muscles are worked hard during a surf session, and stretching them will help prevent bad posture.

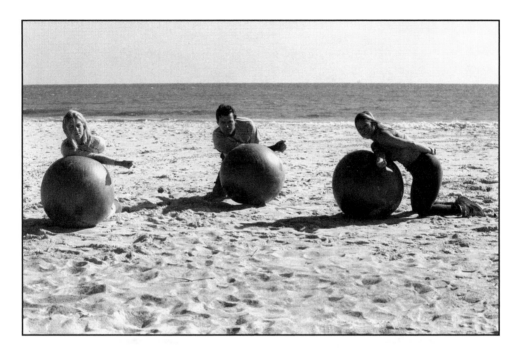

UPPER BACK SHOULDER STRETCH

Place back of arm on the ball and gently press forward. Move your arm at a variety of angles to find and stretch the tight spots. This feels great after a long session in the water. As with all stretches, yoga or Swiss Ball, allow yourself five to ten minutes of stretching. And be sure to stretch before and after each surf session.

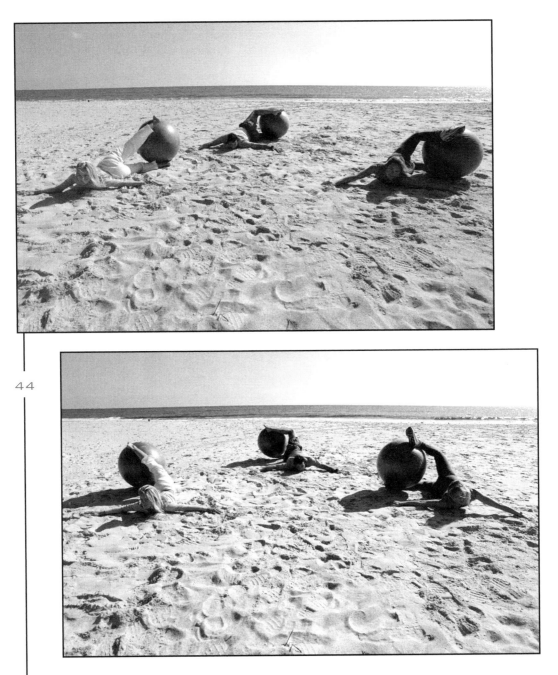

HIP AND LOWER BACK STRETCH

Lie on your stomach, place the ball between your ankles and rotate the ball from one side to the other. Do this in conjunction with the spinal rotation.

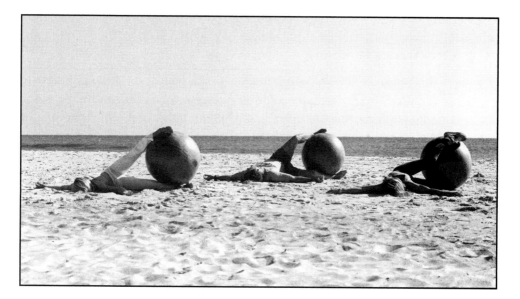

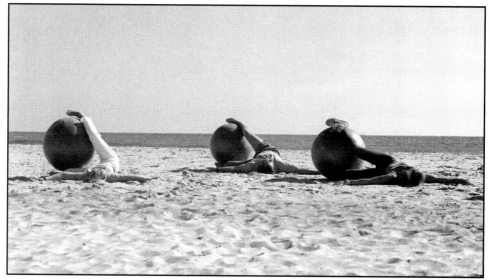

SPINAL ROTATION

Surfing is a rotational sport. Stretching your back and hips is essential. While lying on your back, place the ball between your ankles, and, as you roll the ball in one direction, turn your chin the opposite way. Attempt to keep both shoulders on the ground. You know this is going to feel so goooood!!

THE EXERCISES

The following exercises are effective, practical and fun. Although pre-sented by body part, all exercises incorporate multiple muscle groups, enhance core stabilization, and challenge the body to establish and restore balance. Most importantly, these exercises will help improve your surfing performance.

CHEST/SHOULDERS

The following Swiss Ball exercises promote greater shoulder stability, core strength and balance. A pushing motion is emphasized.

- *Push-ups with legs on ball*
- *Push-up on ball*
- *Leg tuck press*
- *Single leg tuck press*
- *Pike press*
- *Single leg pike press*
- *Dumbbell flat bench press*
- *Dumbbell incline bench press*
- *Dumbbell decline bench press*

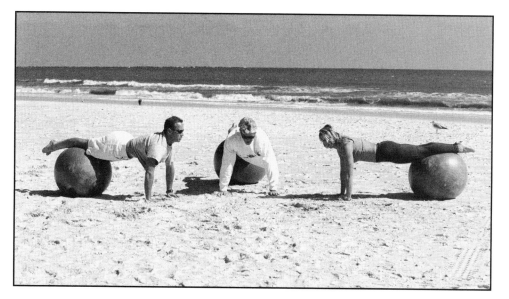

PUSHUPS WITH LEGS ON THE BALL

Fall forward, with your hands on the floor in front of you and your feet on the ball. Do 20 push-ups. The further the ball is from your hips, the harder the push-up. Do not allow your back to sway. Advanced: Do push-ups with only one leg on the ball, alternating legs.

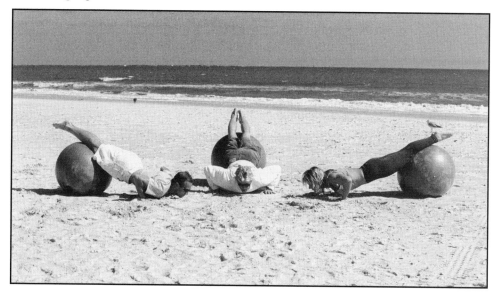

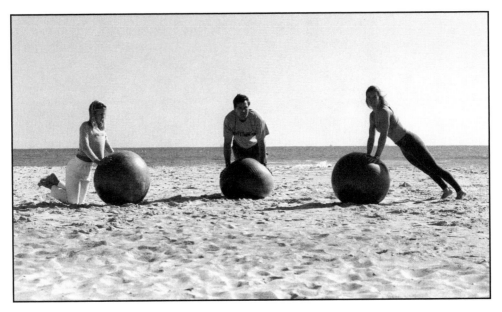

PUSH-UP ON THE BALL

Place hands on the ball and feet behind you in a push-up position. The closer your feet come together, the more challenging the exercise. Lower yourself until your chest touches the ball. Beginners can start with knees on the ground. This exercise works the entire body and strengthens the stabilizing muscles of the torso. These push-ups can be made progressively harder by narrowing your feet position. For a more advanced push-up, support yourself on one leg.

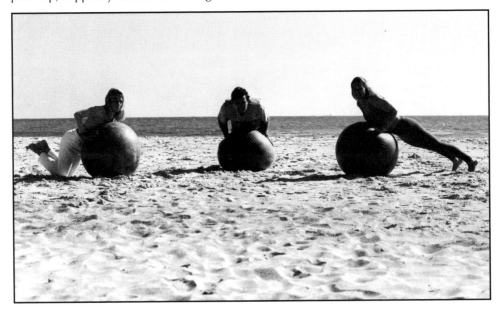

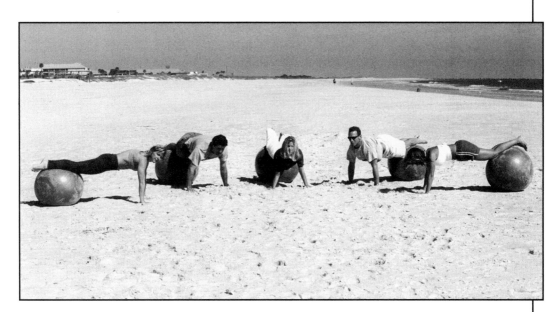

LEG TUCK PRESS

Keep your knees on the ball. In a push-up position, bring your knees to your chest, rolling the ball underneath your lower legs. Pull your abs to your spine. Roll the ball back out again. Do 25 reps.

49

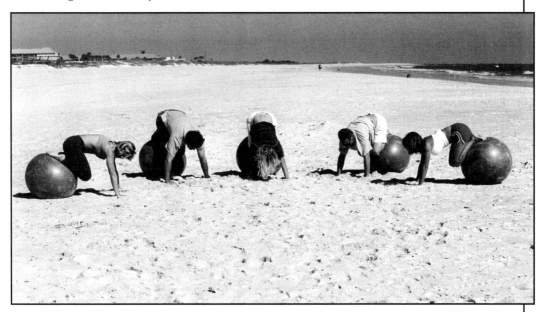

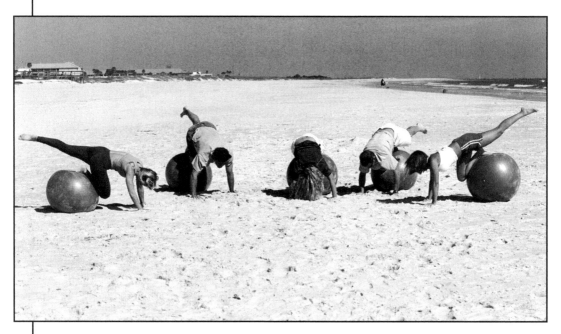

SINGLE-LEG TUCK PRESS

Try the same exercise as the previous one, but use only one leg to roll the ball forward and back. Do 10 reps, then switch legs. This is an advanced exercise.

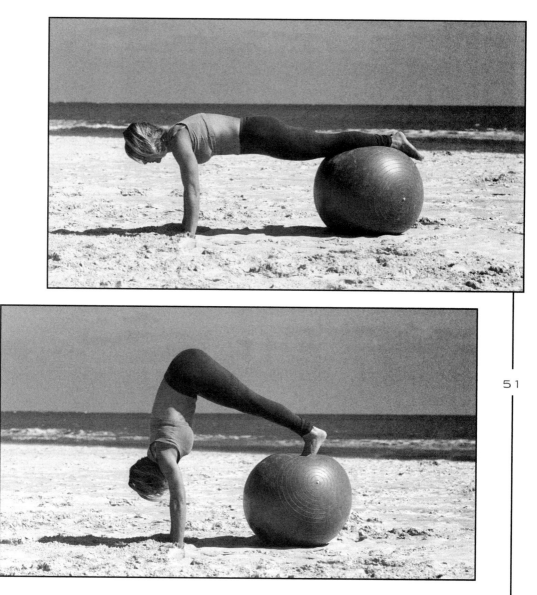

PIKE PRESS

Place your shins on top of the ball, and position your hands beneath your shoulders in a push-up position. Be careful not to dip your lower back. Contract your abs and roll the ball up to the top of your toes. This is an excellent overall body exercise. If you're a real hero, try alternating this move with a push-up.

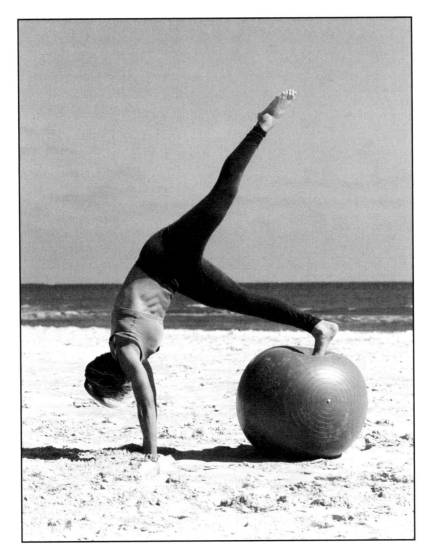

SINGLE-LEG PIKE PRESS

Did you have your Wheaties today? From the finish position of the previous exercise, raise one leg off the ball. Marian Hunter, Surf Sister of the Sea, shows us how it's done! You go, girl! Need I say this is a very advanced exercise? Unless you have abs like these, don't try it!

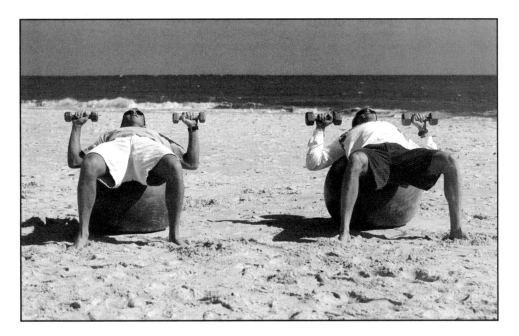

DUMBBELL FLAT BENCH PRESS

Lie with the ball resting under your upper back, your knees bent, and your feet flat on the floor. Hold dumbbells at chest level, and do 20 chest presses, raising the dumbbells straight up toward the sky and lowering again. Make sure to keep your hips elevated, and head relaxed on the ball.

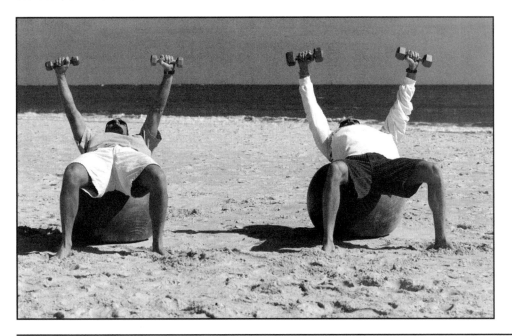

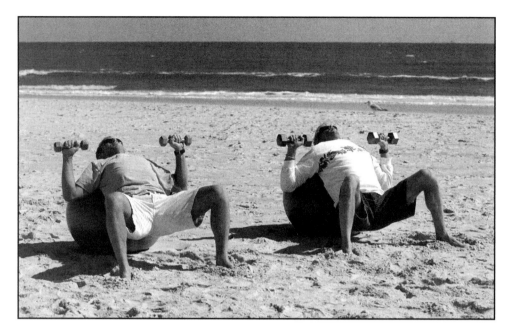

DUMBBELL INCLINE BENCH PRESS

Repeat the chest press again, only roll slightly forward so that the ball is under your shoulders to work the upper chest. Your upper body is now angled as if you were on an inclined bench.

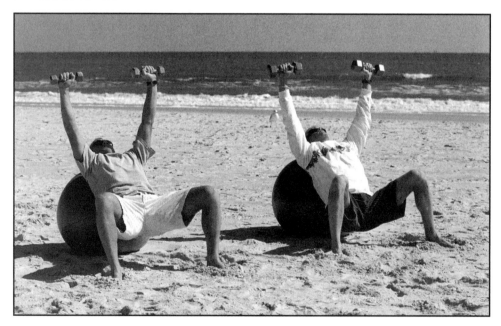

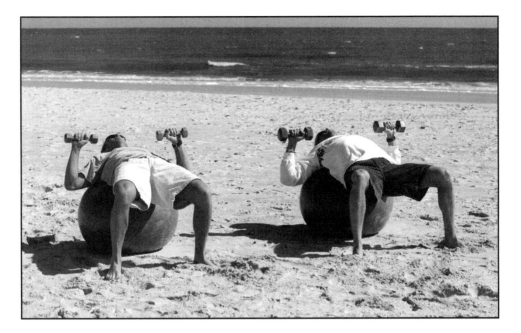

DUMBBELL DECLINE BENCH PRESS

Repeat the chest press, only roll slightly backward so that the ball is under your middle back to target your lower chest muscles. Your upper body is now angled as if you were on a declined bench. Chest presses done at different angles train different areas of the pectoral muscles.

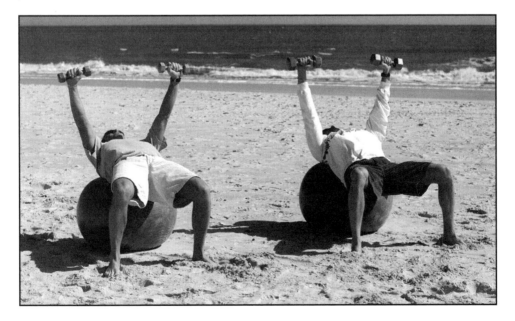

BALANCE

The following exercises are designed to provide balance and stability. Remember, because of its unstable nature, all Swiss ball exercises are core and balance exercises.

- *Surfing progression level 1*
- *Surfing progression level 2*
- *Surfing progression level 3*
- *Surfing progression level 4*

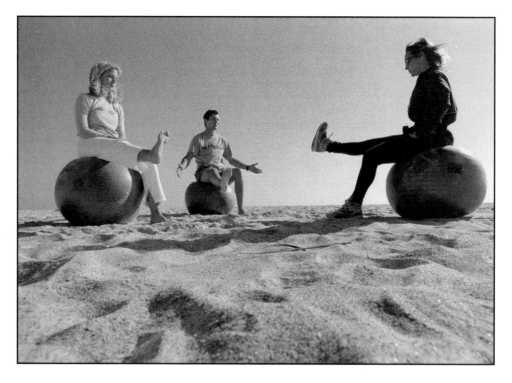

SURFING PROGRESSION: LEVEL 1

Sit on the ball in neutral spine position, with both feet on the ground. Lift one leg and hold for 3 to 5 seconds. Repeat with the opposite leg. This exercise forces you to use your abdominal muscles and your back muscles for balance.

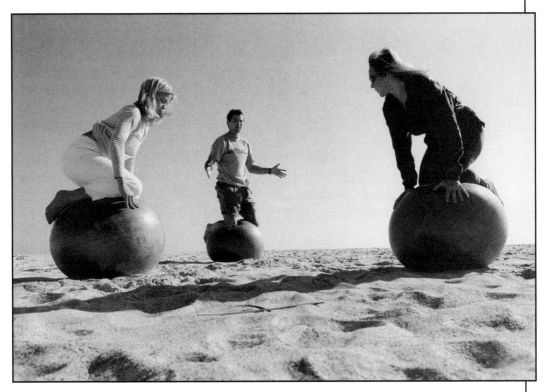

SURFING PROGRESSION: LEVEL 2

Balance with your knees and hands on the ball for 30 seconds.

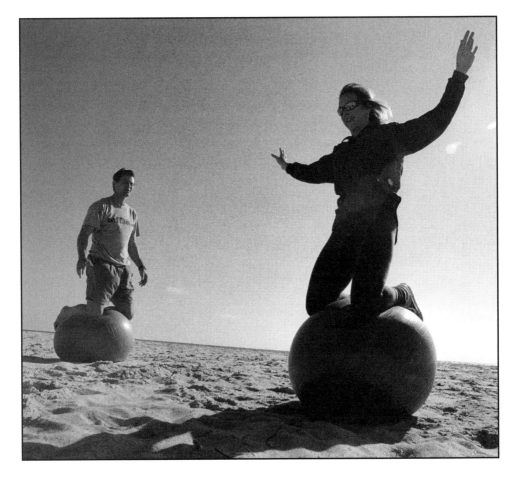

SURFING PROGRESSION: LEVEL 3

Balance on your knees on the ball for 30 seconds. This posture will engage your hips, glutes, lower back and abdominals. Did someone say core strength?

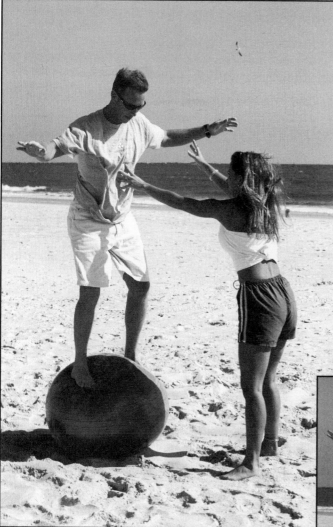

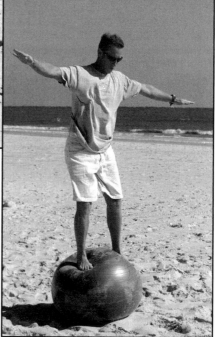

SURFING PROGRESSION: LEVEL 4

Stand on the ball and simulate surfing moves.
My hero Buddy Evans! Don't try this without
proper spotting. This is extremely advanced,
and can be dangerous! If you get this far, and
want an extra challenge, try doing squats.

The purpose of the following exercises is to provide strength to your ventral muscles, namely your rectus abdominus and obliques—the ones that form a rock hard six-pack and stabilize your low back!

- *Sit-ups*

- *Rotations*

- *J strokes*

I began kayak surfing four years ago. My early outings rarely lasted longer than an hour and a half. Sitting on the kayak during the winter surf off of the northern California coast required a constant balancing act. My equilibrium began to improve after integrating the Swiss ball into my daily workout routines. This increased my core strength allowing me to eventually double my time in the surf. I currently work on the ball four to five days a week. I have incorporated balance, stretching and weight training exercises all specific to the Swiss ball into my workout. During this last winter, I was regularly able to surf double sessions totaling six to seven hours. Both over the age of 50, my long boarding partner and I workout regularly to enjoy the ocean and maintain our ability to "hang" with much younger surfers.

—*Enrico Frediani*

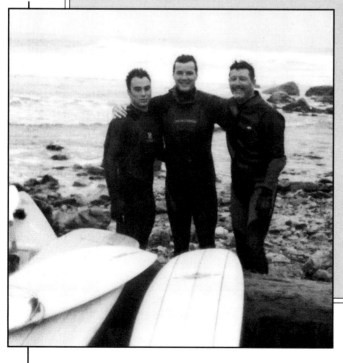

THE AUTHOR (CENTER) IS FLANKED BY HIS SON PAOLO (LEFT) AND HIS BROTHER ENRICO (RIGHT).

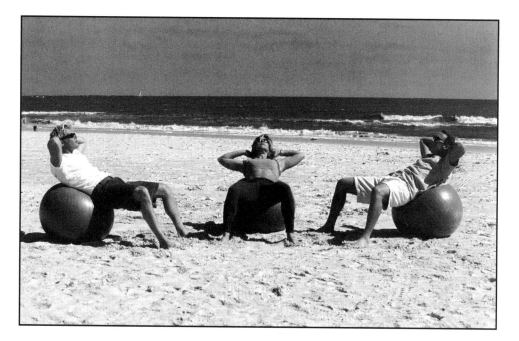

SIT-UPS

Lie with the ball beneath your upper back, your hands behind your head, and your legs bent at the knee. Sit up, crossing your right shoulder to your left knee and then your left shoulder to your right knee. Exercising the obliques (the side of the waist) is very important for trunk stability.

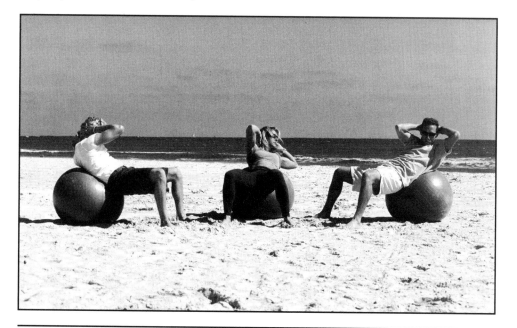

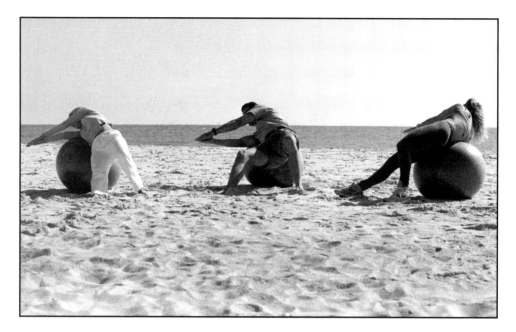

ROTATIONS

Place your lower back on the ball, put your hands together over your chest, and rotate your torso from one side to the other. Placing a weight in your hands will make this an ab strengthening exercise—a real stomach burner!

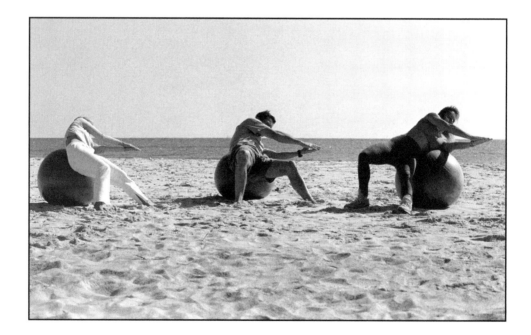

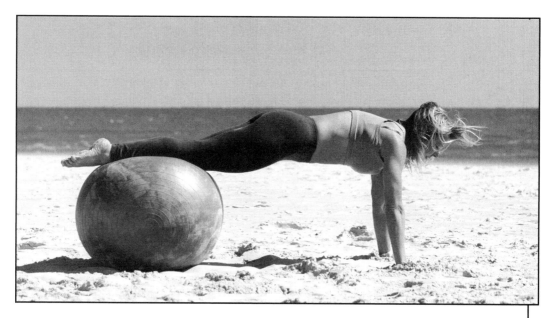

J STROKES

If you fall forward, with your knees still on the ball, use your hips to roll the ball forward and to the right side, back, then forward and to the left side. This is an advanced oblique exercise. Do 25 reps.

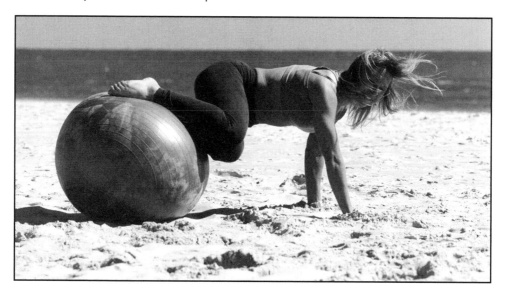

The following exercises are designed to provide leg and hip strength, while effectively improving your balance.

- *Butt blasters*
- *Hamstring curls*
- *Single leg hamstring curls*
- *Single leg lunge*

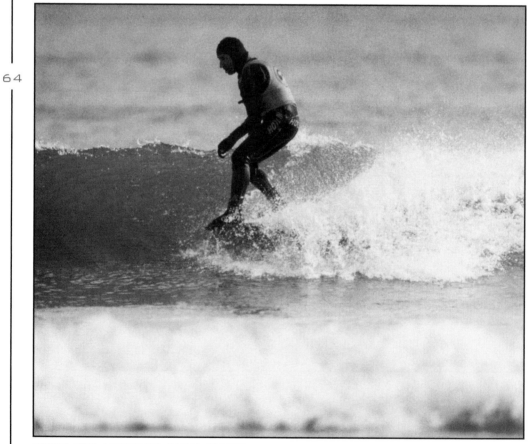

PETER PAN. PHOTO BY JOE McGOVERN.

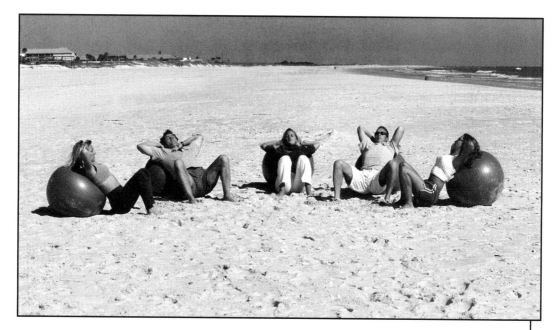

BUTT BLASTER

With the ball under your shoulders, hands behind your head, and feet on the ground, raise your hips and hold for 3 seconds. For a greater challenge, raise your hips while one leg is extended. This will engage your butt, hamstrings and lower back. Stop doing this exercise if it hurts your back.

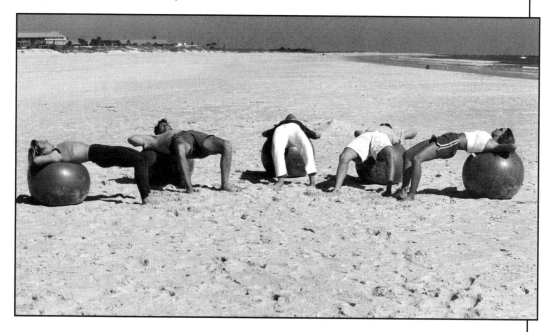

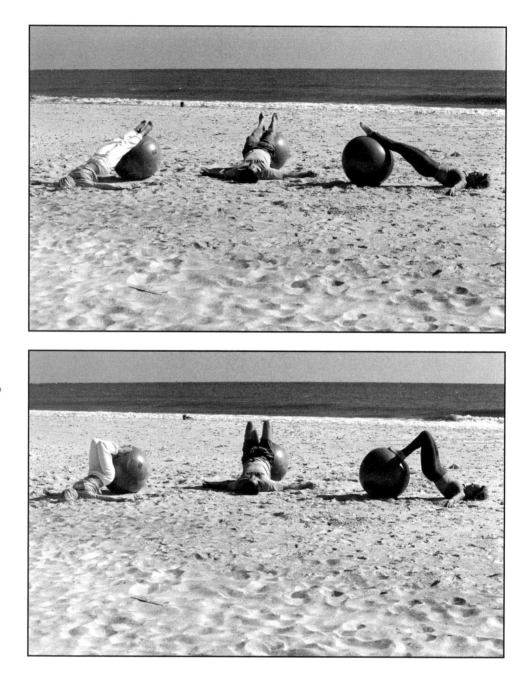

HAMSTRING CURLS

Lie on your upper back with your ankles and calves on the ball. Keep your hips raised, as shown. Keeping your feet on the ball, roll it toward your butt and back out again. For a more challenging workout, try these with your arms folded across your chest.

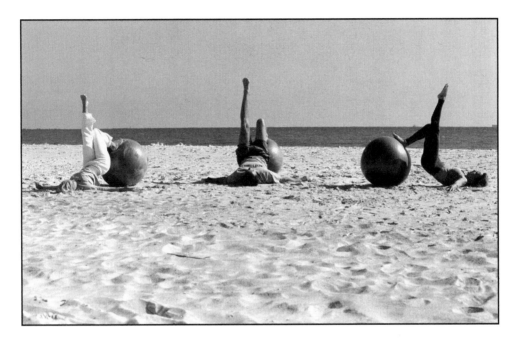

SINGLE-LEG HAMSTRING CURL

Perform the same exercise only with one leg—keep the other leg fully extended, as shown.

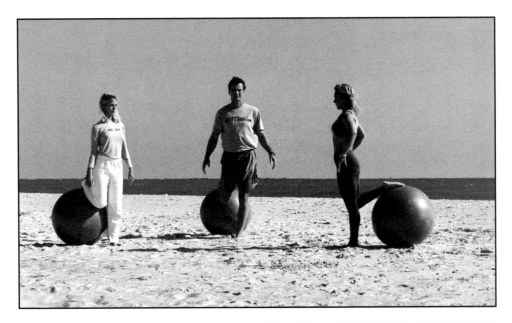

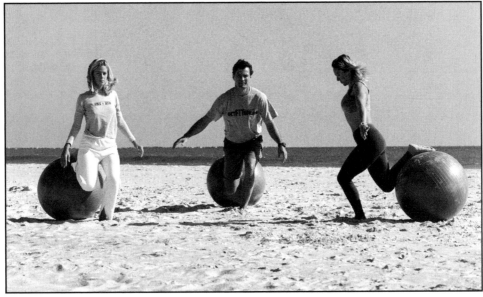

SINGLE-LEG LUNGE

Lunges are great—they're one of the best overall exercises for your legs and butt. They are even better, though, when they challenge your balance. Place your rear foot on the ball and bend your forward leg. For a more advanced version, place only the toe of the your back foot on the ball. Hold weights in your hands to increase intensity. Challenge yourself by reaching your hands to the ground.

The following exercises are designed to strengthen your back and shoulder muscles. A pulling motion is emphasized.

- *Side to side rolls*
- *Contra lateral supermans*
- *Hypers/Arm haulers*
- *Reverse hypers*
- *Rollouts*

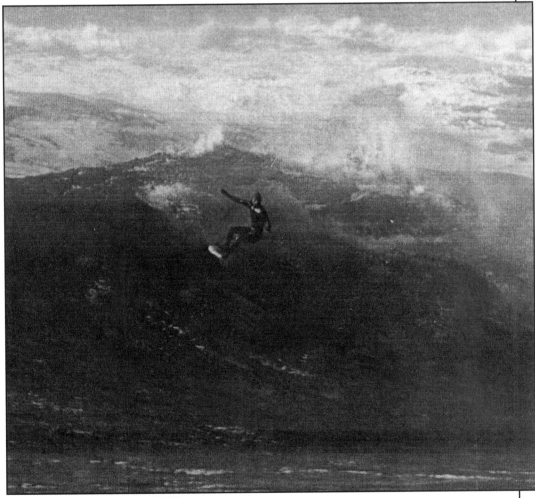

CHARLES DEFAY ON THE EDGE.

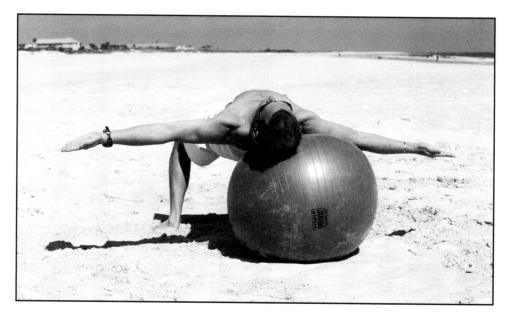

SIDE-TO-SIDE ROLLS

Place your head and top of your shoulders on the ball. Keep your hips well elevated at all times. Roll from one shoulder to the other, pressing the supporting shoulder into the ball. The further away from the center of your body you move, the more intense the exercise. This is an important exercise for surfers as it will counterbalance overused muscles in the front of your body.

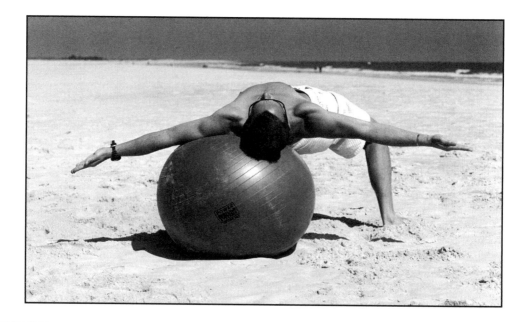

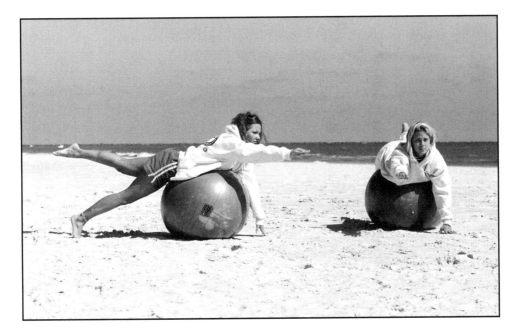

CONTRALATERAL SUPERMANS

Roll forward off ball so that the ball is underneath your abdomen. Alternate lifting one arm and one leg 10 times. Advanced: Roll forward and place both hands on the floor. Lift both legs off the floor.

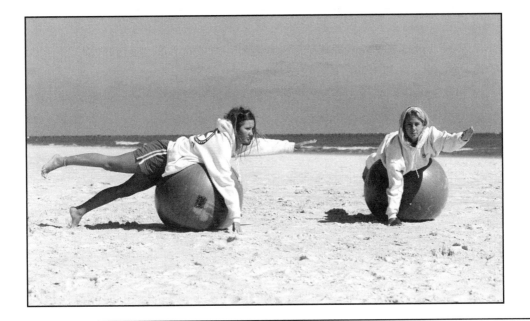

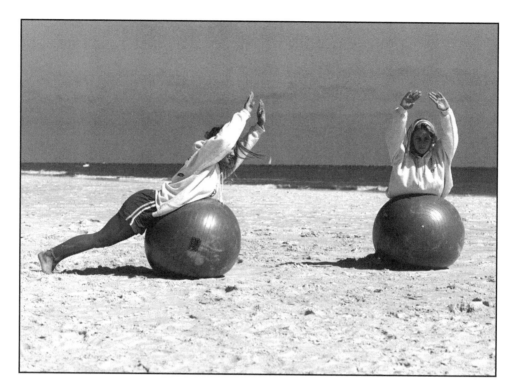

HYPER/ARM HAULERS

Place chest on ball and do 50 arm haulers (see page 97). These help strengthen your paddling muscles. With your arms outstretched in front of you, raise your arms together, to about ear height, and move your hands to your butt and back. Keep your chest high. Advanced: Lower and raise your head as your arms move to your ears. Be careful not to hyperextend your neck.

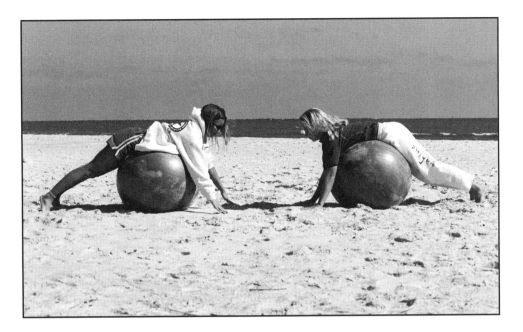

REVERSE HYPERS

Advanced: In the same starting position as the previous exercise, lean forward so that your chin nearly touches the ground. Raise your legs, then lower, but do not allow your knees to touch the ground between reps. Do 15 reps.

73

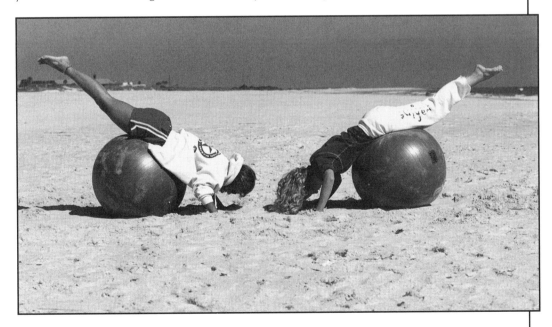

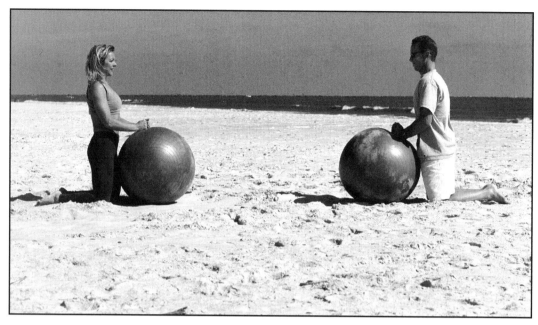

ROLLOUTS

If you fall backward, with your knees on the ground in back of the ball, put your hands together on the ball, and using your elbows, roll forward until your legs are straight and resting on your toes. Do 25 reps. Modify your range of motion if you feel stress in your lower back.

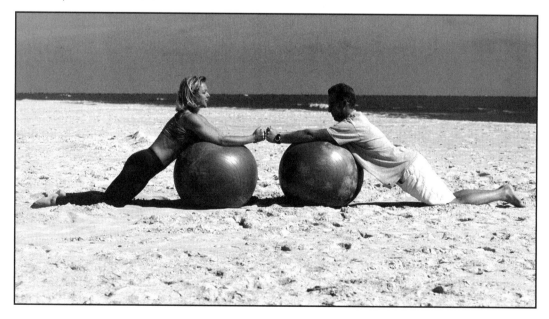

"GO SURFING"

In each Surf Flex workout there is an important balance component. When you see the words, "GO SURFING," try to balance on the ball for at least one minute. Assume any of the following positions in the four-level surfing progression, from beginner to most advanced.
The surfing progression is as follows:
- Level 1: sitting on ball, one foot elevated
- Level 2: kneeling on ball, hands on ball
- Level 3: kneeling on ball, knees only
- Level 4. standing on ball, feet only (spotter present)

Gradually try to progress over time. Challenge yourself by alternating legs (level 1), moving your arms (level 4), and even by closing your eyes!

THE WORKOUTS

Surf Flex combines Swiss Ball exercises to provide a total body workout. The following pages provide you with three workouts (beginner, intermediate and advanced), comprised of the exercises presented in the previous chapter. Perform each workout as a sequenced circuit (i.e., all eight exercises one right after another). Performing one to three circuits of 10 to 20 repetitions for each exercise can serve as a general guideline.

However, volume of training will depend on the skill and fitness level of the trainee, so more reps may be appropriate. Also, dumbbells

Deb Killmon is a highly respected NYC physical therapist, strength and conditioning specialist and certified personal trainer. Deb's five-year service as a senior physical therapist, specializing in cardiopulmonary and orthopedic rehabilitation with New York Presbyterian Hospital, has fashioned her as an invaluable asset to the health and fitness industry today. Deb believes "focus, dedication and consistency equals results!" She is committed to her clients and takes pride in helping them achieve realistic health and fitness goals. For further information Deb can be reached at www.GOTHAM GLOBAL FITNESS.com.

can be added to exercises for greater intensity; much like any weight training exercise performed in a gym setting. If using weights, use lighter loads to ensure safety and proper form. Also, be sure the weights are cleared from your training area when performing balance exercises.

Okay, enough talk, let's do it!

BEGINNER

The following program is designed to introduce you to Swiss Ball training. Perform one to two circuits of 10 to 15 repetitions for each exercise.

- Push-ups (knees on ball)
- Knee tucks
- Half supermans
- Hypers/Arm haulers

- Butt blasters
- Hamstring curls
- Sit-ups (on ball)
- "GO SURFING!"

INTERMEDIATE

This program is appropriate for those who have mastered the beginner routine. It is definitely more intense, since you have a smaller base of support and a larger distance between support points. Perform two to three circuits of 10 to 15 repetitions for each exercise.

- Push-ups (hands on ball)
- Single leg tuck press
- "GO SURFING!"
- Side to side rolls

- Reverse hypers
- Single leg hamstring curls
- Rotations
- "GO SURFING!"

ADVANCED

This workout is the most intense, and requires superior balance and core strength to perform safely and effectively. Progress slowly—it's challenging! Perform three circuits of 10 to 20 repetitions for each exercise.

- Dumbbell presses (flat, decline, incline)
- Pike press
- "GO SURFING!"
- Single leg pike press

- Rollouts
- "GO SURFING!"
- Single leg lunge
- J strokes
- "GO SURFING!"

4

CARDIO CONDITIONING

I practice meditation in the form of "clearing the screen," i.e., erasing all images and inner voices. This helps to keep me relaxed and focused when I'm surfing. It's especially important to stay focused and not to panic when being held down by the force of large waves. Breathing exercises can also help surfers stay calm and focused.

—Tom McBride

Surfing is essentially an interval activity. Surfers physically push themselves to paddle through the waves, and then, once outside, they have the opportunity to recover. The quicker the recovery, the sooner the surfer can choose another wave.

Recovery time is dependent on the surfer's cardiovascular condition—in other words, how efficiently the heart pumps blood throughout the body. Cardio conditioning trains the heart to work more efficiently. Your cardiovascular condition is measured by how many beats per minute your heart is pumping during any given exercise. The fewer the beats, the more conditioned the heart.

The best way to determine your current cardio condition and create a workout that will safely improve it is to determine and monitor your target heart rate. Since surfers come in all ages and fitness levels, heart rate training is an optimal and simple way to monitor and increase the intensity of your personal workout as you get stronger. The

AEROBIC EXERCISE is exercise that uses the aerobic energy system. Aerobic means "with oxygen". This form of exercise includes activities of lower intensity and longer duration such as slow running, long paddling (reef breaks), swimming or cycling.

ANAEROBIC EXERCISE—The anaerobic energy system is used by your body for higher intensity, shorter duration activities such as sprinting through the impact zone. When you're training at 85 to 100 percent of your heart rate zone, you will be operating at an oxygen deficit level. Your body can only tolerate short periods of time at this level. Training at this level will increase your muscles' tolerance to large amounts of lactic acid, and it will improve your ability to sprint hard and fast with a shorter recovery time.

heart is a muscle that can be over- or undertrained—heart rate training will keep you in the proper zone, whatever your age or fitness level.

The simplest way of monitoring your heart rate is with a heart rate monitor. (Polar has very good and inexpensive models.) Otherwise, you can find your heart rate by taking your pulse at your wrist, counting beats for 15 seconds, then multiplying the number of beats by four, for beats per minute. (To find your resting heart rate, discussed below, take your pulse for one minute on three consecutive mornings before getting out of bed, then use the average of the three rates.)

You want to train at your target heart rate, which is 70 to 80 percent of your maximum heart rate. To determine your maximum heart rate (MHR), subtract your age from 220. To determine your target heart rate (THR), multiply your MHR by .70 (for 70 percent intensity) and .80 (for 80 percent intensity). Here is an example for a 35 year old:

MHR = 220 – 35   = 185 beats per minute
THR = 185 x .70 = 130 beats per minute
THR = 185 x .80 = 148 beats per minute

Another target heart rate calculation, known as the heart rate reserve or Karvonen method, takes into account your resting heart rate (RHR):

[(MHR – RHR) x percent of exercise intensity] + RHR

Here is an example of a 35 year old's target heart rate, calculated using the Karvonen method:

MHR = 220 – 35   = 185 beats per minute
RHR = 60 beats per minute

THR = [(185 – 60) x .70] + 60 = 147 beats a minute

Whichever method you decide to use, begin with the low training range (60 to 70 percent of MHR). If you haven't done much weight-bearing or cardiovascular exercise, you'll find that your heart rate will quickly skyrocket. Stay at the lower end of intensity (60 percent of MHR) until your body adapts.

INTERVAL WORKOUTS: ON THE BEACH

The following cardio interval workouts are meant to be done on the beach, with a partner. How often you train depends on your intensity. But bear in mind, most mortals should not train at an anaerobic level, which is 90 percent of one's maximum heart rate, more than twice a week. However, bear in mind that most people should not train at an anaerobic level which is over 90 percent of their maximum heart rate on a daily bases. Your heart is a muscle and like other muscles, it needs time to recover after an anaerobic workout.

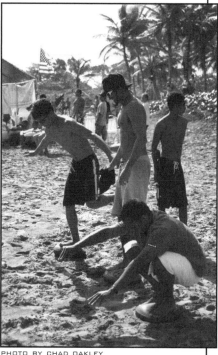

BEGINNER'S CARDIO WORKOUT 1

Go for a light 10-minute jog on beach, then a 3-minute body surf or swim, then another 3-minute jog. Go easy, keeping your heart rate no higher than 70 percent of your max. This is the workout you want to begin with if you haven't worked out for a while and are just getting back to an exercise routine. Repeat 6 times.

PHOTO BY CHAD OAKLEY

BEGINNER'S CARDIO WORKOUT 2

Warm up with a light jog on the beach for 10 minutes. Then, pick up the pace until you're working at 70 to 80 percent of your heart rate. Run into the water and swim beyond the breakers and back in to shore again. Run again for 6 minutes. Keep pace at 70 to 80 percent of heart rate. Repeat these intervals 6 times. Depending on how far the waves are breaking from shore, the swim should also last 6 minutes. This 45-minute workout can be very challenging.

HOT FOOT WORKOUT

This workout is ideal on a wide beach. Start at the beginning point of the soft sand. Run at moderate pace into the water, swim past the breakers (or 3 minutes out), swim back to shore, then run back to the beginning point. Repeat the cycle 6 times. Keep a water bottle handy at the starting point for rehydration.

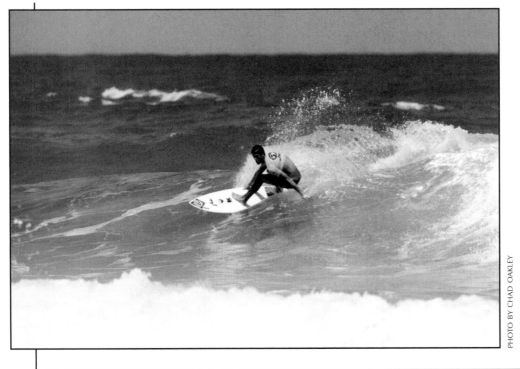

PHOTO BY CHAD OAKLEY

There was a time when most all surfers were excellent watermen. They had to be, out of necessity. Years ago surfboards had no leashes—you lost your board, you swam. More and more surfers today depend too heavily on that leash. Unfortunately, if one snaps, as they often do, you can find yourself in peril. Learning to swim should be a prerequisite and not just a couple of laps at the local pool but at least a mile. Doing so can only increase your confidence and conditioning.

Swimming doesn't have to be tedious. Changing strokes, speed, distance and using hand paddles, fins, kickboards, and buoys can keep these workouts fresh. Work up slowly to the one-mile length, adding one-tenth of distance per week. Try swimming two to three times a week.

Using the kick board, swim one lap kicking freestyle, one lap kicking side stroke, and one lap kicking backstroke. Then do seven laps freestyle, repeat three times, and finish with three laps breaststroke and three laps backstroke. It's a good idea to incorporate plenty of backstrokes. The backstroke helps stretch your shoulders and balance the muscles in your upper body. To get a weekly swimming workout, go to www.swim2000.com.

81

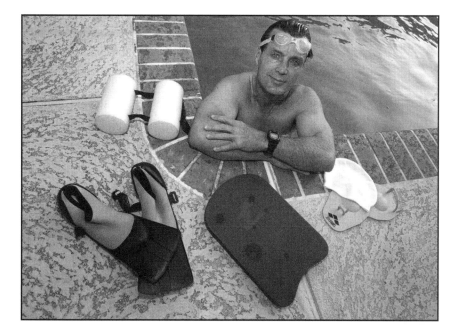

SURF FLEX ASKS STEW SMITH,
FORMER U.S. NAVY SEAL:
WHAT IS HYPOXIC TRAINING?

"The word 'hypoxic' means low oxygen. Adapting this type of training to your swimming workouts is easy, yet it will probably be the most challenging cardiovascular exercise you will ever do.

"Hypoxic swimming easily compares to high-altitude training. Basically, your body is performing with less oxygen because of controlled breath holds while you surface swim. Instead of breathing every stroke or every other stroke, you hold your breath for up to 10 to 12 strokes at a time.

"You will experience increased lactic acid levels, muscle fatigue, and an extremely high heart rate from hypoxic swimming, just as you would if you were running in the mountains. This gets your body used to performing with less oxygen, resulting in increased endurance when you swim regularly and breathe during every stroke. It also increases the length of time you can go without breathing, which can be life-saving if you're trapped underwater after a surfing mishap."

—Stew Smith, former U.S. Navy SEAL and author of *The Complete Guide to Navy SEAL Fitness* and *Maximum Fitness—The Complete Guide to Navy SEAL Cross Training* (Hatherleigh Press)

HEART THUMPER WORKOUT

Running in knee-high water drastically increases the intensity of your workout. Vary the intensity of this workout by changing the depth of the water you run in. Run in ankle-high water for low intensity and knee-higher water for high intensity, getting your knees out of the water and running on the hard sand for recovery. Work your heart rate to 60 to 90 percent of maximum, and repeat so that you've reached 90 percent 6 to 8 times.

ADVANCED WORKOUT 1

Only well-conditioned and competent swimmers should attempt this workout. One partner swims beyond breakers and treads water while the second partner waits 100 or more yards from the water. When the swimmer waves, the runner sprints to the water and swims to his partner. Once he reaches him, he remains treading water while his partner swims back to the starting point. Repeat 6 times.

ADVANCED WORKOUT 2

One partner paddles the surfboard out while the other swims beyond the breakers. Once outside, the paddler can either catch a wave back in or paddle in while your partner remains treading water. The partner with the board paddles out and they switch positions. The partner on the board surfs or paddles in and back while your partner remains treading water. Repeat 6 times.

Most beach communities sponsor open ocean swims. These are great opportunities to maintain your fitness and develop comfort while swimming in the ocean. Another fun way is to body surf. There is no better way to get a better understanding of the waves while getting in ripped shape.

WORD OF CAUTION: ANY WORKOUT THAT IS DONE IN THE OPEN OCEAN CAN BE VERY DANGEROUS. RESPECT THE OCEAN, AND KNOW YOUR LIMITATIONS. DO THESE EXERCISES ONLY WITH A PARTNER AND WITHIN SIGHT OF A LIFEGUARD.

IS CROSS TRAINING IMPORTANT
FOR SURFERS?

"I thought I was in pretty good shape. I surfed a couple of hours everyday, rode the exercise bike for 10 miles 5 days a week, and did a number of sit-ups, push-ups, and leg lifts daily. But in the middle of a competition, I found out—the painful way—the importance of cross training.

"After catching a long left that I rode all the way in, I glanced at the long paddle back, and the endless lines of waves coming in. I opted to run the 50 yards down the beach and jump into the channel. That move probably saved me around 5 minutes, but it trashed my legs.

"Having already been winded from the adrenaline of the heat and the long wave I had just caught, the short jog sucked all the oxygen from my legs and rather instantly made them feel as though I had run a marathon the day before. For the rest of my heats, my turns were only half of what they could've been, my legs felt too weak to push it, and, to make matters worse, I kept falling in situations where I should have easily been pulling my maneuvers. I couldn't figure it out. I wasn't feeling sick, I had got plenty of sleep the night before, I was eating good food all day, yet my legs were giving out on me.

"Later, I talked to my doctor, and he explained how running—using muscles slightly differently than how I was used to exercising during the heat of competition—had effectively zapped my strength and oxygen. To tell the truth, I was pretty zapped for the whole next week. That's when I learned the importance of doing all sorts of different training and strengthening exercises. You never know what kind of muscles you just may need some day. Now I try to perform a mix of exercises."

—Sunshine Makarow,
www.girlsurflife.com

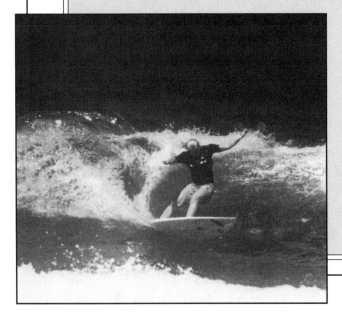

Here are four one-mile swims, based on the standard lap-pool length of 35 meters.

1 Swim 3 laps (back and forth being one length) on the kickboard doing a front kick, then swim 3 laps freestyle, 3 backstroke, 3 breaststroke, 3 sidestroke (alternating side each lap), then 3 backstroke. Repeat 3 times, then finish with 6 laps freestyle.

2 Swim 3 laps easy freestyle, 3 breaststroke, 3 backstroke, and 3 sidestroke. Repeat 3 times.

3 Using the kickboard, swim 1 lap kick forward (chest on the board), 1 kick side (side on the board), 1 kick back (upper back on the board), then 7 laps freestyle. Repeat 3 times, then finish with 3 laps breaststroke, then 3 laps backstroke.

4 Swim 10 laps freestyle, 10 laps with buoy and hand paddles, 10 freestyle with fins, 3 sidestroke, then 3 breaststroke.

SKIPPING YOUR CARDIO WORKOUT

When you can't find a pool or the ocean conditions are too rough, try skipping rope instead. Skipping rope is an excellent form of cardiovascular conditioning, and it really helps develop nimble feet. Here are a few moves that you can easily build into a routine.

When skipping rope, focus on how your feet land and the deceleration of the downward momentum as your legs catch your body weight. Land softly without making a thumping sound with your feet. Keep shoulder relaxed. The rule is *one rotation of the rope, one skip!*

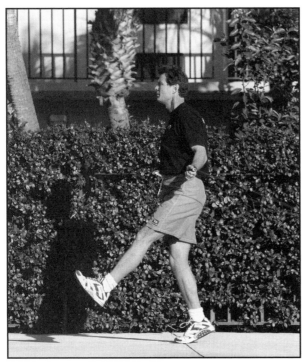

In kickout skipping, kick one leg out between skips. For more intensity, bring your knee to your chest. This exercise will strengthen your abdominals.

Finally, try crossing your feet every other jump. This move is great for your inner and outer thighs.

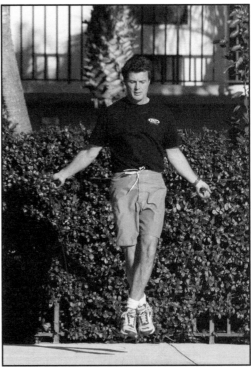

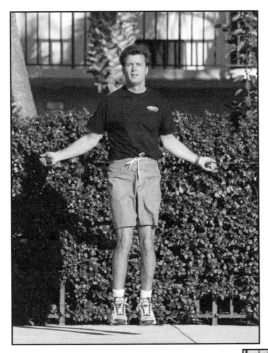

In standard rope skipping, both your feet jump simultaneously.

In this variation, try alternating feet as you skip.

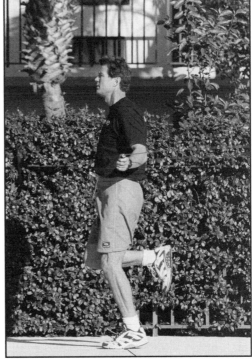

WHAT'S YOUR SECRET
TO MAINTAINING CARDIO FITNESS?

"The easiest way to keep in shape for surfing is to surf as much as possible, on all kinds of boards, in all kinds of conditions, regardless of how pathetic the waves are. I do this all winter (so I have many days of surfing by myself). I try to wear the heaviest wetsuits I can find, so I get a good workout. I treat every session as a run, and try to keep paddling and catching waves.

"When there is no surf, I go to plan B, which is to work out either by teaching or taking Tae Kwon Do and cardio kickboxing classes several times a week. I began Tae Kwon Do in 1979 and have never stopped. This is probably the best thing I have ever done to help my contest surfing and free surfing. Because of all the stretching and flexing in the martial arts, I can stay flexible, even at my advanced age of 50. Tae Kwon Do and kick-boxing are highly aerobic, so they give you big lung capacity for surfing hard.

"When I don't do that, plan C is running, which I have done since high school. I ran distance and varsity track in both high school and all four years of college. I have noticed that overrunning has ruined many athletes, so I try not to overdose on it.

"For me, the key to keeping in good surfing shape is to always be ready to surf in a contest. There is always one not too far in the future, so I make myself work out to be ready for it."

—Peter Pan, one of the first inductees into the East Coast Surfing Hall of Fame; first surfer from New England to place in a professional contest (O'Neill Pro-Am); only surfer from the Northeast to have a signature surfboard model on the West Coast (Hobie Peter Pan Slug Model—a top seller for about six years); only surfer to ever place in international competition from New England (Festival of Surfing, Noosa Head, Australia); recently placed in five finals at the 1999 ESA Northeast Regional Surf-Offs (Open, Grandmasters, Senior Longboard, Senior Bodyboard, and Kneeboard), winning the Professional Longboard Association East Coast Championships for five straight years, and taking sixth place in the Legends Final at the Noosa Longboard Festival.

5

WHEN IT'S FLAT:
DRY LAND WORKOUTS

You might be wondering how dry land training could improve your surfing. How does running, jumping, pulling and pushing exercises improve surfing skills? A better-conditioned athlete is the athlete that has that extra edge which makes him succeed where other athletes fail. What cross training will do is make you a better athlete and provide much needed rest to the overused and overworked muscles that you have developed while surfing. It will also reduce the risk of injury that is associated with muscular imbalances by allowing the tendons, bones and connective tissues used in your primary sport to rest.

While conditions may not always be optimal for surfing, there is no excuse for not keeping in shape. Using your own body weight is one of the most functional and oldest forms of exercise. Most of these exercises are multi-joint and multi-plane. This means that you are using more than one joint per exercise (a bicep curl, for instance, is only a one-joint exercise) and moving your body through several ranges of motion (backward, forward, side to side and rotational). This type of training will keep your body strong, flexible and agile. Not only will it maintain your body's ability to move in a full range of motion, it will also develop the strength and power a surfer needs in their ever-changing field of play—the ocean.

High impact workouts (plyometics) will also train your body to absorb the shock of big drops and floaters. It will condition your legs and hips to stabilize and decelerate under your full body weight. Being able to do so will not only help you avoid knee injuries, it will help you stabilize quicker in critical situations so that you can set up your next move.

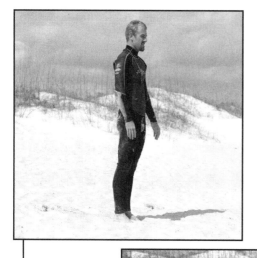

8-COUNT BODY BUILDERS

From a standing position, squat down, placing your hands on the ground (that's 1). Kick your legs back so that you're in a push-up position (that's 2). Spread your legs out wide (3), then bring them back together (4), bring your chin down to the floor (5), push up again (6), bring your legs back to the squat position (7), then return to standing position (8). Do 10 times.

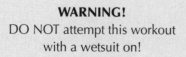

WARNING!
DO NOT attempt this workout
with a wetsuit on!

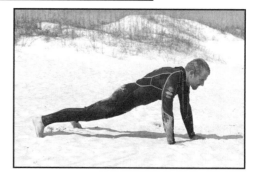

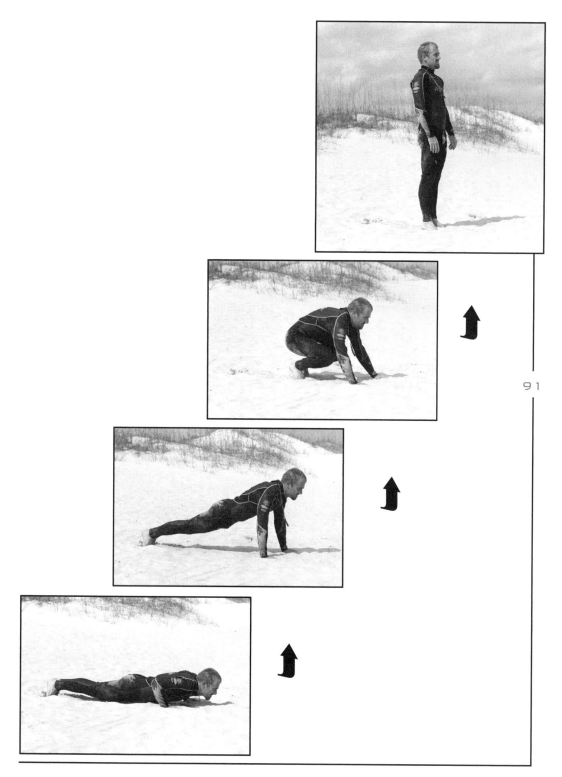

WHEN IT'S FLAT: DRY LAND WORKOUTS

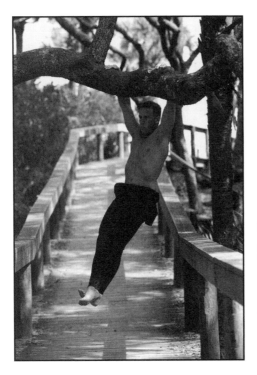

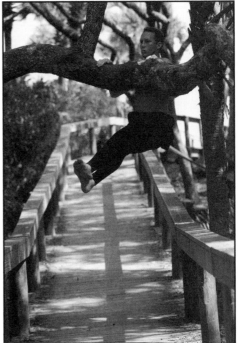

PULL-UPS

The wider the grip, the harder the pull-up. Start with a wide grip and do 2 pull-ups; then swing around the bar and do 2 pull-ups with a reverse grip; then swing back to the other side and do 2 more pull-ups with a narrower grip. Repeat the sequence, ending with wide-grip pull-ups.

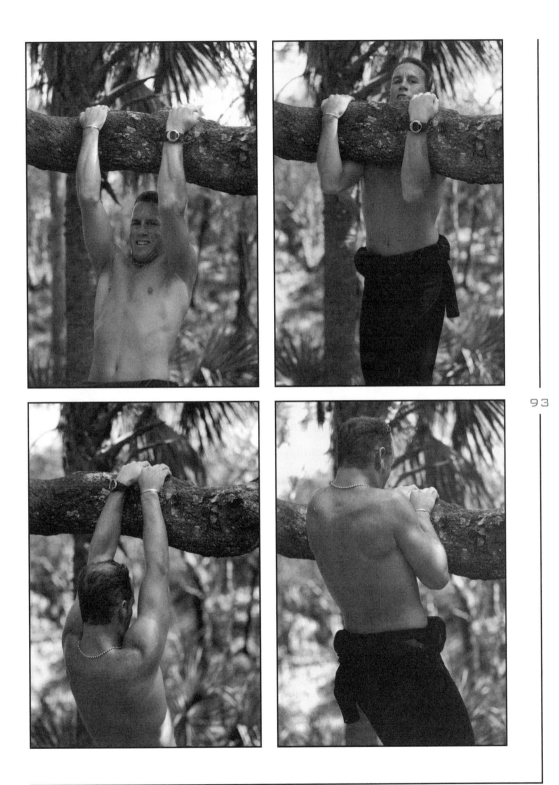

WHEN IT'S FLAT: DRY LAND WORKOUTS

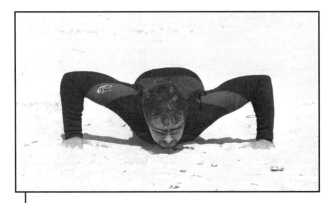

PUSH-UPS

Changing the position of your hands helps to target different muscles. Do 20 push-ups with your arms out wider than your shoulders.

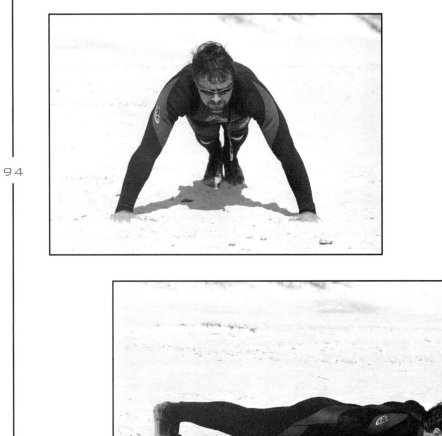

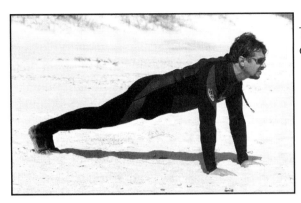

Then do 20 with your arms directly beneath your shoulders.

Then do 10 with one arm out wide in front and the other arm down and to the side, as shown. Do 10 more, switching your arms' positions.

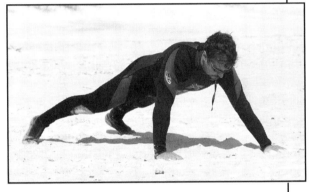

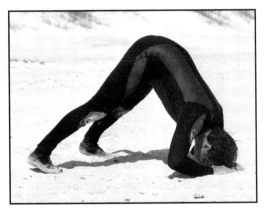

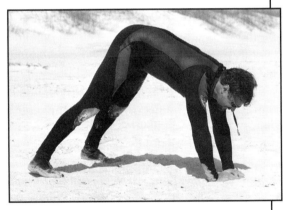

Then finish with 10 Chinese push-ups in which your hands are placed directly beneath your head so that your fingers form a triangle and your hips are raised.

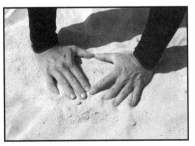

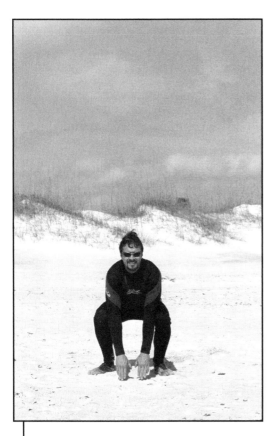

STAR JUMPERS

Stand with your feet shoulder-width apart and squat so that your hands touch the ground. Leap up, getting both feet off the ground and reaching your hands toward the sky. Do 15.

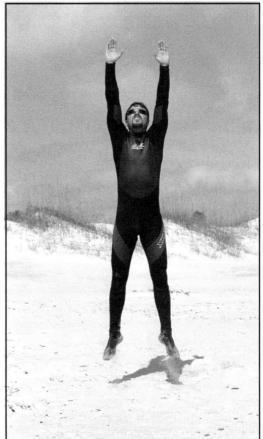

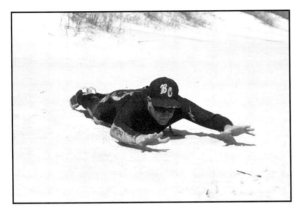

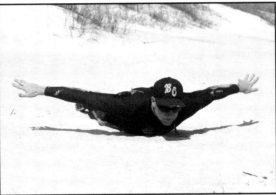

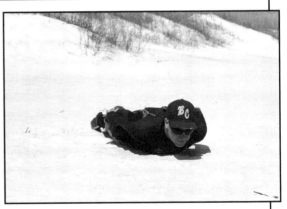

ARM HAULERS

Lie on your stomach with your arms outstretched in front of you. Raise your arms together, to about ear height, and move your hands to your butt and back. Keep your chest high. Do 50.

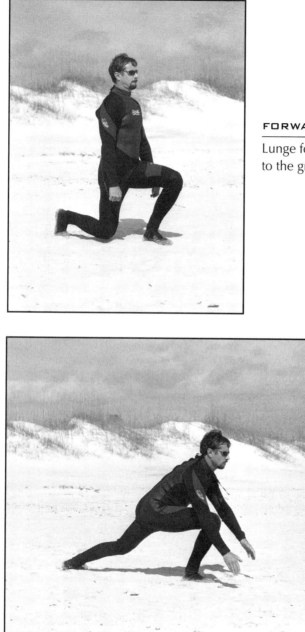

FORWARD LUNGES

Lunge forward, bringing your back knee to the ground. Do 20 per leg.

LUNGE AND REACH FORWARD

As you lunge forward, reach your hands out in front of you. The deeper you lunge and the greater the reach, the more you increase your range of motion and flexibility in your legs, hips and back.

SIDE LUNGES

Lunge to the side, rather than forward. This motion strengthens your inner thigh. Do 20 per side.

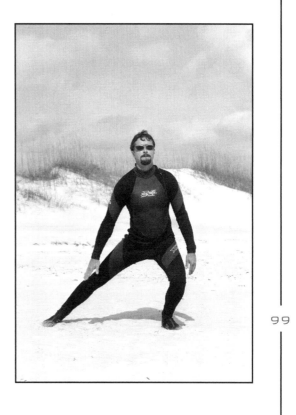

If you want to attain your highest level of performance you better be conditioned. Each sport or discipline has different objectives in the quest for ultimate condition. Certainly a sprinter has different muscle, cardiovascular and other conditioning needs than a marathoner. Surfers who are at the cutting edge of performance must make training and conditioning a conscious part of their lives. Keep surfing and stay happy.

—Fred Hemmings, 1968 world surfing champion and author of *Soul of Surfing*.

RIDING THE MAVERICKS:
FITNESS AT THE EXTREME EDGE OF SURFING

BY GRANT WASHBURN

Surfing is one of the most difficult and physically challenging sports known to man. The unique and unforgiving wilderness of the ocean, combined with the incredible force of breaking waves, provides a playing field unmatched by conventional activities. Surfing a wave of any size takes a remarkable amount of strength, balance, experience, and coordination.

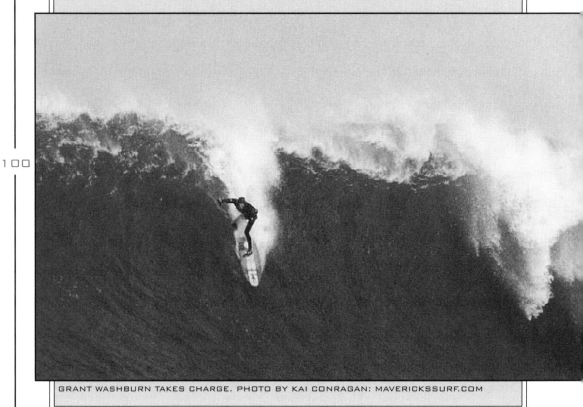

GRANT WASHBURN TAKES CHARGE. PHOTO BY KAI CONRAGAN: MAVERICKSSURF.COM

Many of the physical requirements for surfing are best developed by the act itself, but some are not. A surfer who does nothing to balance the water workouts won't be well prepared, and is far more likely to be injured or to develop serious problems. When the waves get huge, perhaps 40 to 50 feet high, the sport demands an even greater commitment. To safely ride big surf at a place like Mavericks, you need to be more than just a great surfer; you need to be a great surfer with the conditioning of a triathlete. You may be forced to paddle like a powerboat, hold your breath for minutes, then swim for miles, and if you run out of gas it may cost you your life. Big waves raise the stakes, and when you are caught inside by the most terrifying set you have ever seen, it is nice to know you trained your body to deal with the situation.

Despite the dominating power at work, many surfers have enjoyed long careers riding giant waves. Ken Bradshaw and Jeff Clark recently rode the biggest waves of their lives while in their 40s, and they're still surfing strong! Last winter I had the privilege of surfing 12-foot Sunset Beach with Peter Cole, who is nearly 70, and he rode without a leash!

Accomplishments like these continue to redefine surfing, and to inspire people all over the world. Through proper conditioning we can surf bigger waves, better, more often, and for a lot longer than anyone believed possible.

—Grant Michael Washburn has lived on Ocean Beach in San Francisco for nearly a decade, studying and working in film production—and chasing big waves. In the spring of 1998 he completed his first documentary film, *Maverick's*, a personal project detailing the rise of the world's most infamous big wave surf spot. Grant, who has been surfing the giant waves alongside the best in the world, narrates the film he co-directed and produced. With the help of a professional team, including surf legend Jeff Clark, filmmaker Lili Schad, and award-winning writer Bruce Jenkins, Grant was able to capture the essence of the story and to deliver some of the most unbelievable surfing images ever captured. The film was showcased at the Hawaiian International Film Festival and the Sun Valley Film Festival in 1999. Grant is constantly collaborating on new projects, including the Imax film *California* by Greg MacGillivray, *The Endless Summer III*, and a feature film being produced by Tom Hanks.

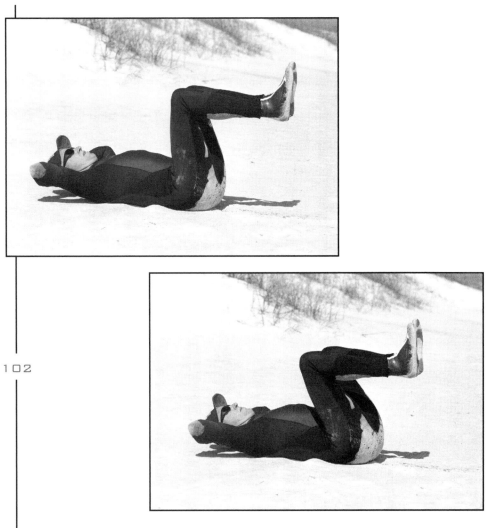

LOWER ABS

Lie on the ground with your hands behind your head. Raise your legs off the ground so that they are bent at the knee. From this starting position, raise your hips slightly off the ground. Do 50.

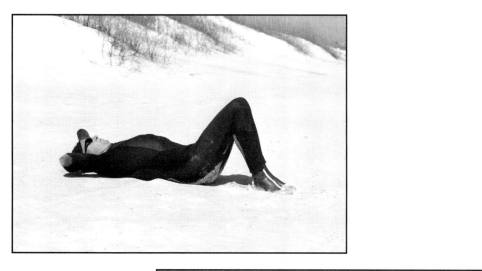

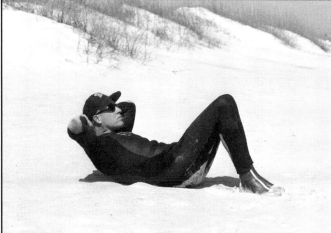

UPPER ABS

Lie on the floor with your hands behind your head, your knees bent, and your feet flat on the floor. Raise your shoulder blades off the ground, lower slightly, then raise again. Do not let your shoulder blades touch the ground between reps. Do 50.

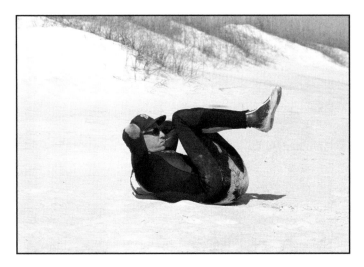

FULL CRUNCH

Lie on the floor with your hands behind your head, your legs elevated, and your knees bent. Raise your shoulder blades off the ground as you bring your knees toward your chest. Again, do not let your shoulder blades touch the ground between reps. Do 50.

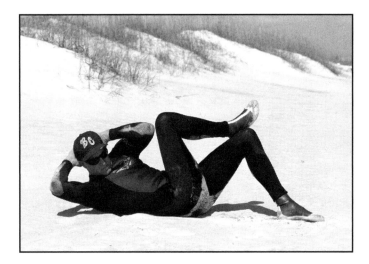

OBLIQUE CRUNCH

Lie on the floor with your hands behind your head and both knees bent. Crunch up so that your left elbow touches your right knee. Do 25, then raise your left knee and crunch to your left side 25 times.

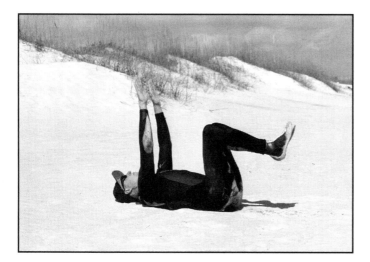

DEAD BUG

Lie on the floor with your arms perpendicular to your body and your legs elevated and knees bent at 90 degree angles. Concentrate on keeping your back firmly pressed into the ground. If your back arches, shorten the range of motion in your legs. As you lower one arm to the ground above your head, lower and extend the opposite leg toward the floor. Return to starting position, and repeat with opposite limbs. Do 25.

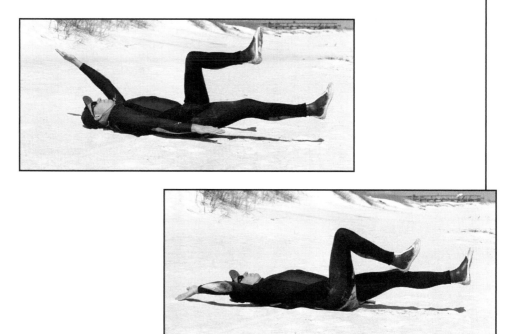

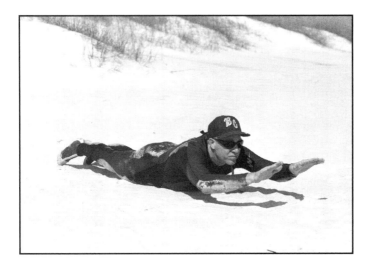

SUPERMAN

Lie on your stomach with your arms and legs fully extended. Raise your arms slightly off the ground, until your chest rises. Keep your legs on the ground. Do 20.

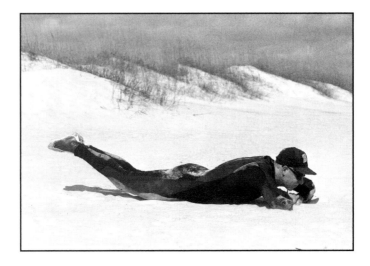

LOIS LANE

Lie on your stomach, bend your knees, and place your chin on your hands, as shown. Raise your thighs off the ground. Repeat 25 times.

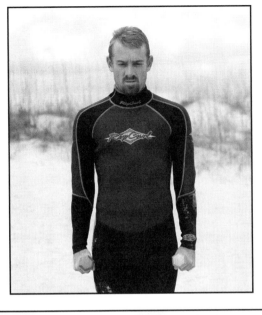

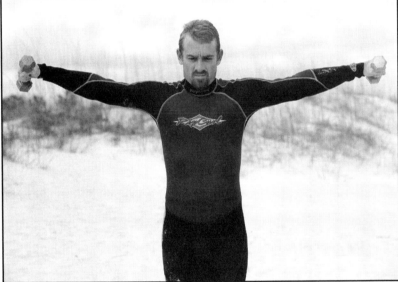

LATERAL RAISES

Hold 2- to 5-lb. dumbbells in each hand at your sides. Raise the dumbbells out and up to the shoulder height. Do 20. Do not lift the weights higher than shoulder-height.

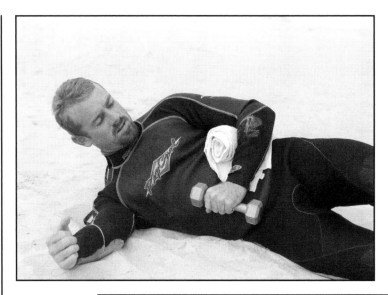

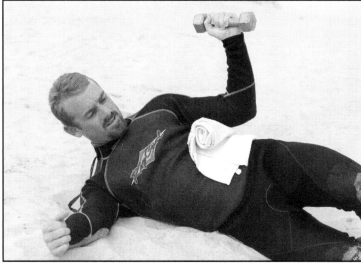

ROTATOR CUFF EXTERNAL ROTATION

Lie on your right side, with a towel under your left elbow. Hold a 2- to 5-lb. dumbbell in your left arm and rotate your forearm from a position parallel to the floor to a position perpendicular to the floor, keeping your elbow on your side. Do 20. Repeat on the opposite side. This exercise is extremely important for maintaining healthy shoulders.

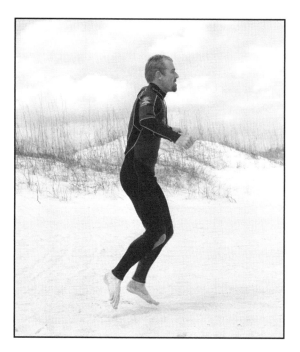

JUMPING SPLIT-SQUATS

Standing in a lunge position, jump and switch your foot positions. Do 15.

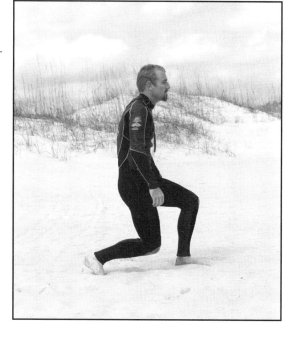

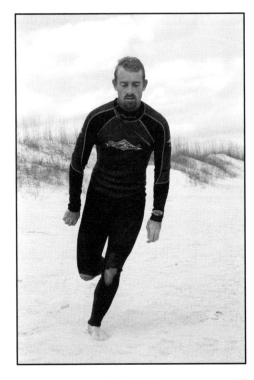

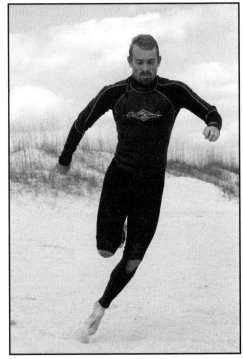

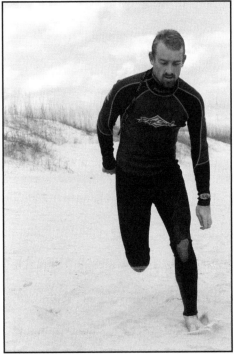

LATERAL LEG HOPS

Stand on one leg and hop across an imaginary line. Do 15 with each leg.

The following workouts are just a guide. You can get as creative as you like. But keep in mind that these might be above or below your current fitness level. You should never increase your reps if your form fails, nor should you attempt to complete either of these workouts if they are too strenuous. Let your form be the indicator as to whether the number of reps you have chosen are correct for you. It's best to do fewer reps with good form than to be wiggling and straining to complete a desired set. Also, never begin a workout with your abdominals. Save these for last. You will need your abdominal strength for maintaining good posture for upper and lower exercises. When you find that you can complete a full set in good form, increase the repetitions by ten percent.

AROUND THE WORLD

 5 Eight-Count Bodybuilders
 5 Pull-ups
10 Forward Lunge (each leg)
10 Push-up
10 Side Lunge (each leg)
10 Wide Push-up
10 Lunge and Reach Forward (each leg)
10 Chinese Push-up
10 Lunge and Reach Side
30 Lower Abs
50 Arm Haulers
10 Jump and Split Squat
20 Superman
15 Single Leg Hops (each leg)
25 Oblique Crunch to the Right
20 Lois Lane
25 Oblique Crunches to the Left
25 Dead Bug

UPPER · LOWER – MIDDLE

UPPER

10 Eight-Count Bodybuilders
 5 Pull-ups
10 Push ups

50 Arm Haulers
10 Eight-Count Bodybuilders
5 Bicep Grip Pull-ups
10 Wide Push-ups
50 Arm Haulers
10 Eight-Count Bodybuilders
5 Wide Grip Pull-up
10 Chinese Push-ups
50 Arm Hauler

LOWER

10 Star Jumpers
10 Forward Lunge (each leg)
10 Side Lunges (each leg)
10 Lunge and Reach Forward (each leg)
10 Lunge and Reach Side (each leg)
10 Single Leg Hops (each leg)

MIDDLE

25 Lower Abs
10 Superman
25 Oblique Right Side
10 Superman
25 Obilque Left Side
10 Superman
25 Dead Bug

THE MEXICAN MILE

Here's a simple anaerobic workout guaranteed to get you top shape. I learned this workout from my old boxing trainer Vic Grupico. When I first got serious about boxing and wanted to compete, I went to see Vic with hopes that he would train me. After the first few weeks of sparing, I discovered that I couldn't go more than a round and a half without being fully exhausted. I was running six miles a day so you would think that I could go three three-minute rounds easily. Vic said that I was doing my roadwork (running) all wrong. He laid out the following workout for me. After a month of this training, I was going four to six hard rounds with the pros.

Go to your local high school track. Warm-up by jogging two slow laps. Then stretch or do a pre-surf yoga salutation for five minutes.

LEVEL ONE—Start by standing at the beginning of the straightaway of the track, then sprint (or run as hard as you can) until you reach the curve. Walk this section of the track. This should give you plenty of recovery time. When the curve ends, sprint the straightaway again. Do this for four laps equaling one mile.

LEVEL TWO—As you get in better condition, and your able to recover quickly during the walking portion, jog the curves instead of walking.

LEVEL THREE—When you become accustomed to level two, incorporate running backwards, shuffle side to side, and lunge walks during the curve portion.

After you've achieved this level, begin to increase the mileage. But don't add junk miles. Two miles should be the max. Think in terms of increasing the intensity of the sprints instead of increasing the mileage. You will love the results of this workout. Not only will you be getting in top shape, you'll discover why sprinters have the best abs in the world.

SECRET AB WORKOUT

This very effective abdominal workout will not only strengthen your abs, it will do wonders for your lower back. And the best thing is that you can do it anywhere. All you have to do is inhale and pull your belly button as tightly as you can in toward your spine. Hold it for five seconds. Then exhale all your breath out and draw your belly button tightly to your spine again, and hold for another five seconds. Repeat this exercise for two minutes. You've just given yourself a great ab workout. This exercise trains the transverse abdominal, the deepest of the abdominal muscles. This muscle is like a girdle around your waist. Keeping this strong is important for your trunk stabilization.

TRICK QUESTION:
DO YOU KNOW HOW TO BREATHE?

We all do it every moment of every day, from the moment we're born. Unfortunately, most of us have forgotten what comes naturally. As we breathe, our diaphragm lowers, giving room for our lungs to expand. If you place your hand below your belly button you should feel an expansion of your belly when you inhale. You can feel the same expansion when placing the palms of your hands on the sides of your lower back. If you don't feel this expansion, you're not breathing correctly.

To see an example of perfect breathing, watch a baby breathing while he's asleep. What you will observe is a full belly and lower back expansion, the chest hardly moving. Most adults are chest breathers, especially athletes. Ask an athlete to take a deep breath and they will most likely suck in their stomach and expand their chest. This does not allow the lungs to expand to their full capacity.

To see if you are a chest breather, place one hand on your chest and the other below your belly button. Breathe naturally. Your belly should expand two-thirds more than your chest. If you're like most adults, you probably don't breathe this way. We've been conditioned to "suck it up"—life's tensions, worries, and stress all contribute to poor breathing. By the time we're adults we've lost the path of our natural breath.

The importance of breathing is crucial when surfing. Proper breathing makes sure our blood is full of oxygen, which we need while holding our breath under water, and it can also save your life if you are caught in a stressful situation.

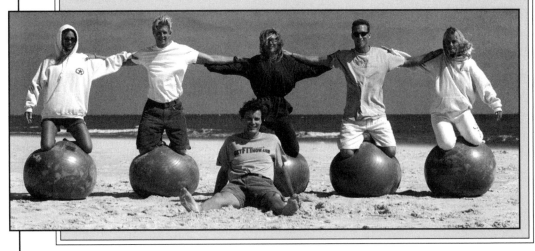

6

THE WAHINE WORKOUT

When I began surfing in the mid-'60s I rarely saw a woman surfing. Where I surfed, in Northern California, most of the time the water was cold and the skies gray—not really *Baywatch* conditions. We used only long-sleeve wetsuits, and it would take a good while to warm back up after surfing by standing around a burning tire. Then my buddies and I would smell so bad of rubber it would take two showers to remove the smell. . . . Surfing was tough and not very glamorous.

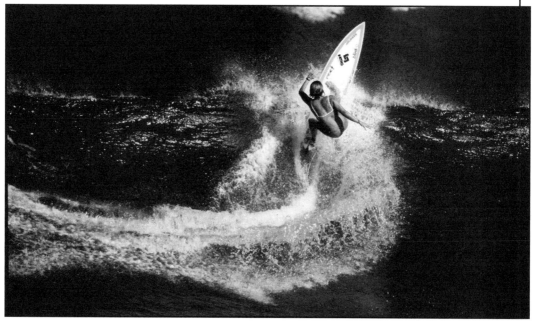

JODI NELSON IN ACTION. PHOTO COURTESY PHOTO: RUSSI.

But I do vividly remember the one female surfer whom I saw consistently in the water. Joan Weston was her name; she was a big, strong, strapping blonde, who also happened to be a roller derby queen. Joan was the captain and chief enforcer for the Bay Area Bombers. I watched her most Saturday mornings on TV while eating my cereal as a kid. She was one tough and athletic lady.

Today, women are the fastest growing segment of the surfing population. And women have their specific sports-related surf issues. The issue that is most quickly recognizable is the lack of upper body strength. During childhood and adolescence, women are not encouraged to develop this strength. Most high school or college sports that women participate in, with the exception of swimming and gymnastics, require strong cardio conditioning but sorely lack any real upper body development. This strength, though, is the foundation of paddling out.

If, like many women, you haven't the foundation of this upper body strength, it is highly recommended you begin a strength training program. It is very important to begin by conditioning your rotator cuffs (shoulders). If you don't, you're looking for trouble down the road. Your upper body muscles will only get as strong as your rotators will let them. Furthermore, if you push yourself before you're ready you can do serious damage to your shoulders. So before you begin this program, let's take a look at a healthy rotator cuff routine.

Surfing is a very physical sport and it is very easy to think that if you are surfing everyday you don't need to do any other form of exercise. I feel this is a common mistake many surfers make. If you do not train or work on strength outside of the water, your surfing skills tend to get stagnant. Working with such great tools as the Swiss Ball, wobble board, and latex band will make an unbelievable difference in strengthening your core muscles and it also improves balance.

As a professional surfer, being paid to do what I love is a dream and I take it very seriously. Being in the best shape both physically and mentally is a challenge, but is the key to success in this sport.

—Jodi Nelson

ROTATOR CUFF WORKOUT

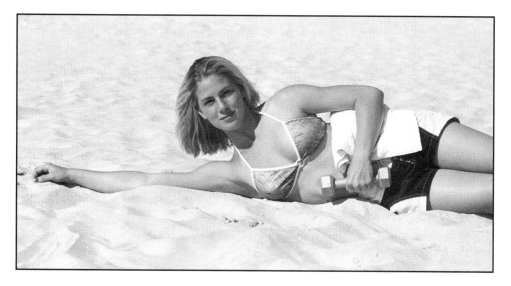

ROTATOR CUFF EXTERNAL ROTATION

Lie on your right side, with a towel under your left elbow. Hold a 2- to 5-lb. dumbbell in your left arm and rotate your forearm from a position parallel to the floor to a position perpendicular to the floor, keeping your elbow on your side. Do 3 sets of 20, resting 30 seconds between sets. Repeat on the opposite side.

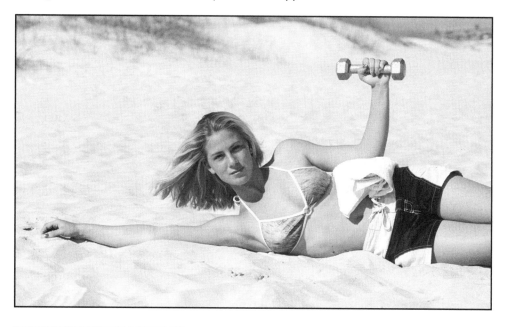

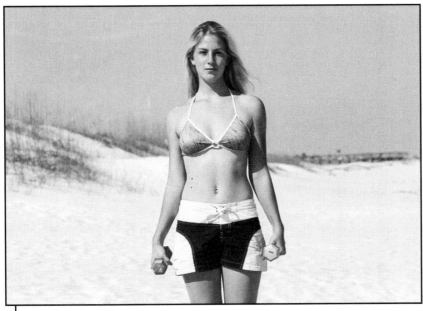

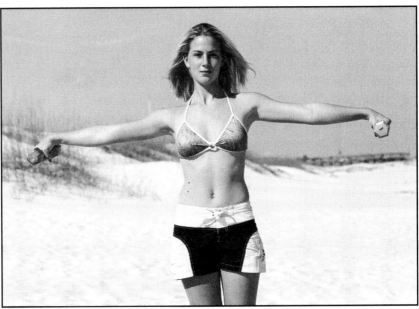

LATERAL (ROTATOR CUFF) RAISES

Kneel or stand on the ground and hold 2- to 5-lb. dumbbells in each hand at your sides. Raise the dumbbells out and up to the shoulder height. Do 20.

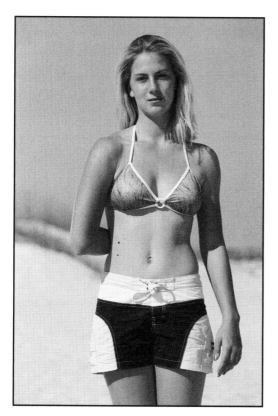

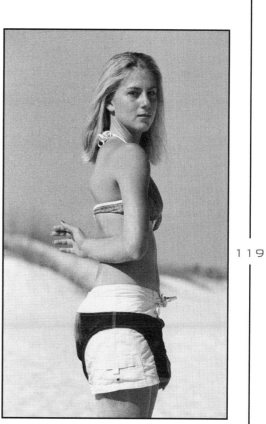

ROTATOR CUFF EXTERNAL ROTATION STRETCH

Place one hand behind your back and press your elbow forward. Repeat on the opposite side.

In a 1999 study, *The American Journal of Sport Medicine* suggested that a well-rounded training regiment of strength training, stretching and plyometics (*see jumping rope, dry land workouts) could prevent 80 percent of female ACL injuries.

It is also noted that most women over-train the front of the thigh (quadriceps). This imbalance can create instability in the knee joint. Strong hamstring (back of the thigh) exercises should be encouraged to balance the muscles of the leg (see p. 66).

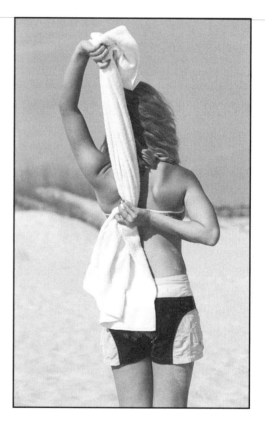

HAND-BEHIND-BACK STRETCH

With each hand holding the opposite end of a towel, place one hand behind your lower back and the other behind your upper back. Raise and lower the towel, as if you're drying your back.

Merchandise presented for return, including sale or marked-down items, must be accompanied by the original Borders store receipt. Returns must be completed within 30 days of purchase. The purchase price will be refunded in the medium of purchase (cash, credit card or gift card). Items purchased by check may be returned for cash after 10 business days.

Merchandise unaccompanied by the original Borders store receipt, or presented for return beyond 30 days from date of purchase, must be carried by Borders at the time of the return. The lowest price offered for the item during the 12 month period prior to the return will be refunded via a gift card.

Opened videos, discs, and cassettes may only be exchanged for replacement copies of the original item.
Periodicals, newspapers, out-of-print, collectible and pre-owned items may not be returned.
Returned merchandise must be in saleable condition.

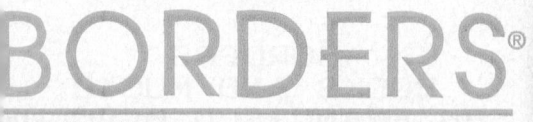

Merchandise presented for return, including sale or marked-down items, must be accompanied by the original Borders store receipt. Returns must be completed within 30 days of purchase. The purchase price will be refunded in the medium of purchase (cash, credit card or gift card). Items purchased by check may be returned for cash after 10 business days.

Merchandise unaccompanied by the original Borders store receipt, or presented for return beyond 30 days from date of purchase, must be carried by Borders at the time of the return. The lowest price offered for the item during the 12 month period prior to the return will be refunded via a gift card.

Opened videos, discs, and cassettes may only be exchanged for replacement copies of the original item.
Periodicals, newspapers, out-of-print, collectible and pre-owned items may not be returned.
Returned merchandise must be in saleable condition.

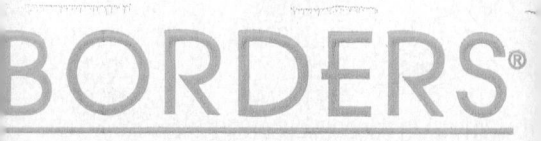

Merchandise presented for return, including sale or marked-down items, must be accompanied by the original Borders store receipt. Returns must be completed within 30 days of purchase. The purchase price will be refunded in the medium of purchase (cash, credit card or gift card). Items purchased by check may be returned for cash after 10 business days.

Merchandise unaccompanied by the original Borders store receipt, or presented for return beyond 30 days from date of purchase, must be carried by Borders at the time of the return. The lowest price offered for the item during the 12 month period prior to the return will be refunded via a gift card.

Opened videos, discs, and cassettes may only be exchanged for replacement copies of the original item.
Periodicals, newspapers, out-of-print, collectible and pre-owned items may not be returned.
Returned merchandise must be in saleable condition.

BORDERS®

Here are descriptions of some of the exercises you'll be doing in the workouts that follow:

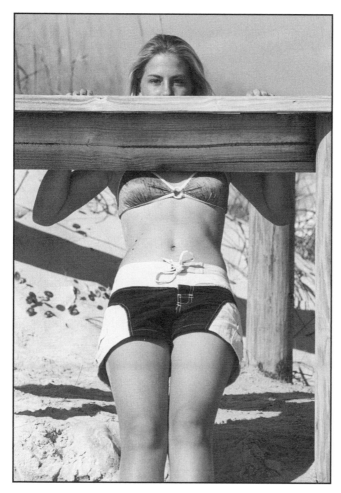

PULL-UPS

Yes, you can do pull-ups! With the proper training any woman can do them. Why don't many women do them? Because they don't practice. The development of a strong latissimus dorsi (that big muscle on the side of your back) will give you the pulling power you need for paddling. If you cannot do a pull-up, try doing a negative. Begin at the up position and lower yourself down slowly for five to eight seconds. It's helpful to do negatives with a friend who can assist you to the up position by placing her hands under your feet or behind your shoulders, and pushing you up.

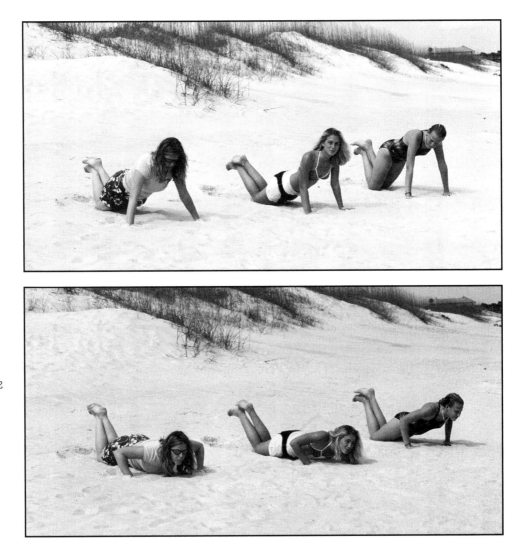

PUSH-UPS

Push-ups strengthen the chest and arms, muscles you need to push yourself into a pop-up and hold your board while duck diving or turtle rolling. They're also a great way to strengthen the abs. If you're not strong enough to do push-ups on your toes, begin by doing them on your knees. Then practice negatives by starting at the top position and lowering yourself slowly to the ground.

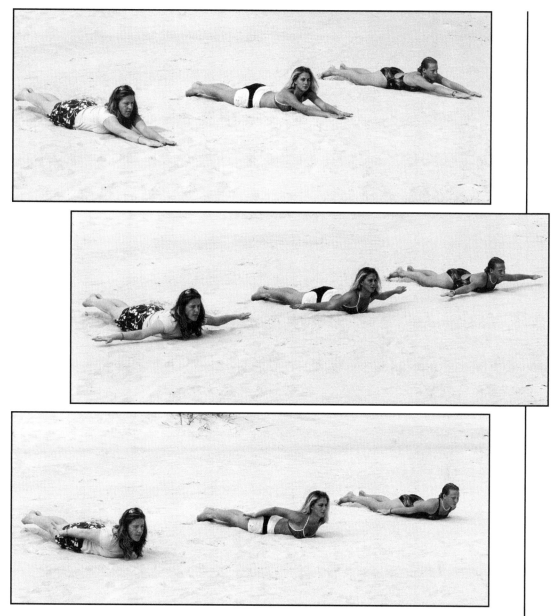

ARM HAULERS

Lay on the ground and place your arms above your head. Squeeze your shoulder blades together, engaging your back muscles, lift your chest and bring your hands down to your hips. Repeat 50 times. Do not allow your hands to touch the ground. Arm haulers and the next exercise, Delt Burners, strengthen the upper back and shoulders. Adding a slight chin tuck and lift will strengthen the back of the neck, which can otherwise become easily fatigued while paddling.

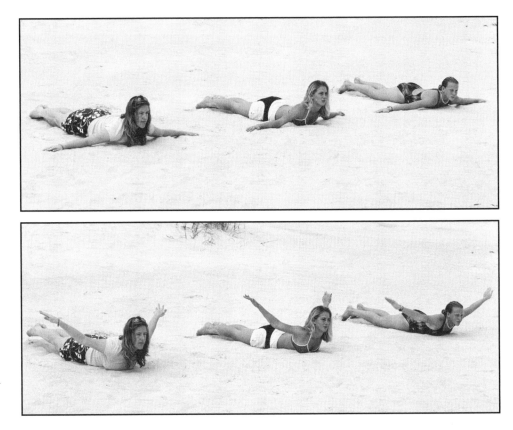

DELT BURNERS

Lie on your stomach with your arms out to your sides, perpendicular to your body. Raise and lower them. Attempt 25 repetitions after you have completed the Arm Haulers.

According to the American Academy of Orthopedic Surgeons, it is important that women get enough calcium to build bones and help prevent osteoporosis (experts recommend at least 1,000 to 1,500 milligrams of calcium a day). Bone loss can start at the age of 35, but can be slowed down with calcium supplementation and weight-bearing exercises like jogging, power walking and strength training.

The following routines incorporate the exercises above. They can be done at a maximum of every other day. Do not train if your muscles are sore. The following combinations of push-ups, pull-ups, arm haulers, and delt burners are meant to hit all the major muscles groups used in paddling. These are not substitutes for the variety of exercises in the Dry Land Workout in the previous chapter, which are necessary to condition your entire body.

Each routine is progressively more difficult, so once you can do one routine with ease, move on to the next.

STARTERS—REPEAT 3 TIMES

- 10 pull-ups on a low bar, with knees bent
- 10 push-ups, on knees
- 10 arm haulers
- 5 delt burners

SPONGER—REPEAT 3 TIMES

- 10 pull-ups on a low bar, with legs straight
- 10 push-ups on knees
- 10 arm haulers
- 5 delt burners

BEACHBREAK—REPEAT 3 TIMES

- 10 leg-assisted pull-ups
- 5 push-ups on toes, then 5 negatives
- 10 arm haulers
- 10 delt burners

POINTBREAK—REPEAT 3 TIMES

- 10 leg-assisted pull-ups, then 2 negatives
- 10 push-ups from toes (if you can't complete 10, do negatives at failure)
- 15 arm haulers
- 10 delt burners

> 10 leg-assisted pull-ups, then 3 negatives
> 10 leg-assisted pull-ups, then 3 negatives
> 10 push-ups on toes
> 15 arm haulers
> 10 delt burners

After completing this section successfully and continuing with your rotator cuff workouts, continue the REEFBREAK WORKOUT once a week and add the following MAVERICKS workout once a week.

MAVERICKS

Try doing four sets of the following routine, resting 30 seconds between sets:

Set #	Pull-ups	Push-ups	Arm Haulers	Delt Burners
1	3	6	15	10
2	4	7	15	10
3	3	6	15	10
4	2	4	15	10

THE Q ANGLE

The Q angle is a problem for athletic women; it is a major source of knee problems. The Q angle is the degree of the outside of the hip to the outside of the knee. Men generally have a Q angle of 10 degrees, women 15 degrees. An increase of the Q angle places greater stress on the knee, which can result in pain and inflammation. Angles of 20 percent or more increase the likelihood that the quadricep will pull the kneecap to the outside causing bad tracking of the knee (patellofemoral pain).

Stretching the outside portion of the leg and hip and strengthening the inner leg muscles can help eliminate this problem. The following exercises will help you.

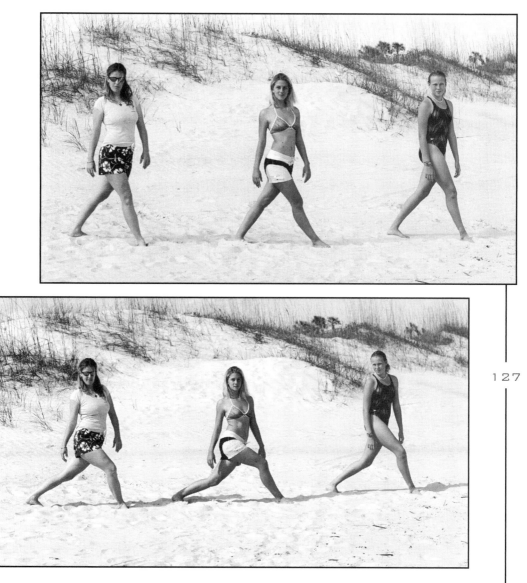

STANDING HIP STRETCH

Stand and step one leg back and to the opposite side. Be sure to keep the heel of the front leg on the ground. Repeat with the opposite leg, stretching the front of your thigh and the hip of your back leg.

According to Sports Illustrated for Women, *"In the past decade, 1.4 million fe-males athletes have suffered ACL injuries." The ACL one of the ligaments in the knee joint that attaches the thigh and the shinbone.*

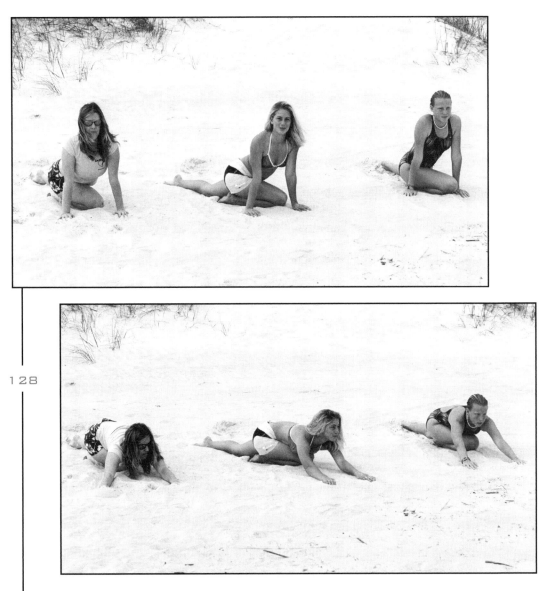

PRONE HIP STRETCH

Lie on the ground with one knee under the opposite side's shoulder. Keep your hands in front of you. Repeat with the opposite knee, stretching the outer hip and the glute of your forward leg.

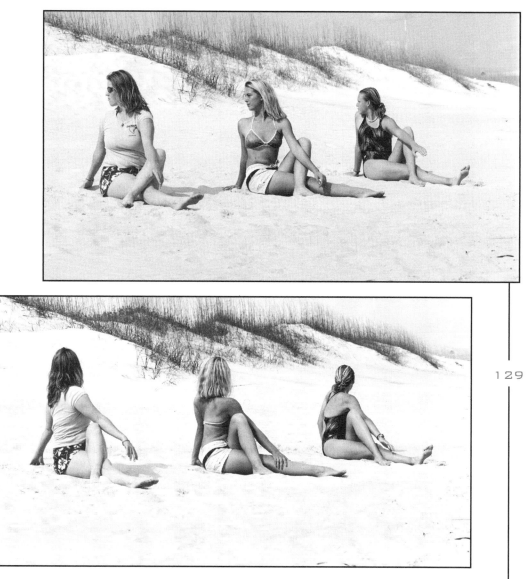

SEATED CORKSCREW

Maintaining good posture is key to this stretch. Sit on the floor with your right leg extended in front of you. Keep your back straight. Cross your left foot over your right leg. Place your left hand by your side on the floor and your right elbow behind your left knee and turn your spine to the left, then to the right. Switch legs and repeat, stretching the outer thigh, hip and torso. Increase this stretch by pressing your forward arm against the outside of your leg.

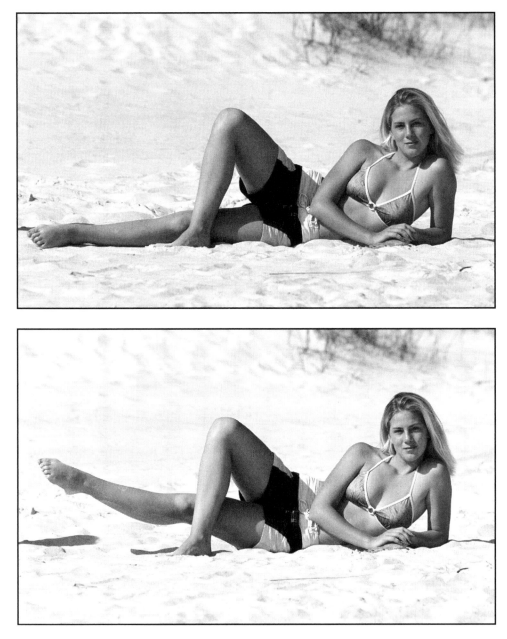

SIDE LEG RAISERS

Lie on one side with the lower leg extended and upper leg bent at the knee and crossed over the lower one. Maintaining strong inner thigh muscles is important for knee stabilization. Repeat on the opposite side.

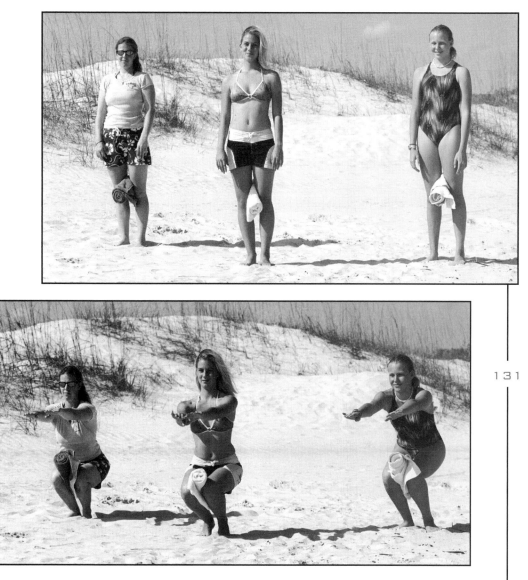

SQUATS WITH TOWEL

Stand with a towel between your knees. Squat while squeezing the towel. Repeat 20 times. Strengthening the vastus medialis (the small muscle of the inner thigh near the knee) will help keep your kneecap tracking properly.

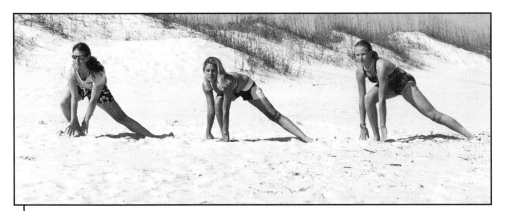

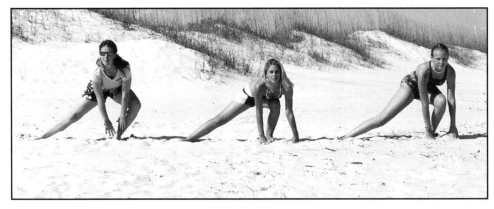

ALTERNATING SIDE LUNGE

Lunge from one side to the other. This exercise stretches and strengthens your inner thighs.

STRETCHING AND STRENGTHENING WORKOUT

Standing Hip Stretch—five times per leg

Prone Hip Stretch—three times per leg (hold for 10 to 20 seconds)

Seated Corkscrew—two times on each side (hold for 10 to 20 seconds)

Side Leg Raises—three sets of 25 per leg

Squats with Towel—three sets of 25

Alternative Side Lunges—20 times on each side.

SURF FLEX ASKS DONNA PLOURD, RN, FNP:

WHAT COMMON AILMENTS DO YOU TREAT FEMALE SURFERS FOR?

"Women athletes often complain of thigh and/or knee to shin pain, which is most intense after activity. The pain or ache subsides after periods of rest. It is commonly attributed to the shortened tendons of women's legs. Avoiding the problem is simple—stretch! Specifically, stretch the thigh by bending the knee.

"In my practice I also see a lot of what we call 'surfer's ear.' It's a fungus that grows in the ear, common to surfers or swimmers who experience prolong moisture in the ear canal. Symptoms include ear pain, ear discharge, muffled hearing, and other similar problems. One way to avoid it is to make sure you dry your outside ear well with a towel or use a blow drier to gently blow into the canal for five minutes.

"After 20 years of surfing, I've found that even a week away from it can affect your ability to paddle with strength and endurance. Staying in shape for that next long day in the lineup is always on my mind. A friend, who is also a pro surfer, introduced me to swimming on those off days. It's the closest thing to surfing that you can simulate and it has worked well for me."

—Donna Plourd, RN, FNP is the third generation of women surfers in her family. After 22 years of surfing, longboarding is in her blood. She is a Family Nurse Practitioner, who works in a clinic at a local beach town in San Diego. She also maintains a Web site that focuses on the average female surfer, Water Wahine at:

members.aol.com/surferdp/surferdp.htm

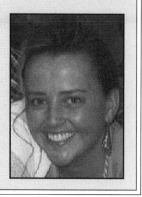

SURF TO LIVE; LIVE TO SURF

BY GERRY LOPEZ

I remember hearing that soccer and motocross were the two most strenuous sports, but the people who made that determination never considered paddling out at the Pipeline on a 10-foot day. They also didn't consider the fact that paddling out was about the same as arriving at the beginning of the soccer game or the start of the motocross race. In surfing, the race doesn't really begin until after you make it out to the line-up. It's then you face the danger of getting caught inside in the take-off zone where the waves are biggest. Perhaps you work up the nerve to attempt a ride where, if you don't make the drop, you will certainly get pounded into the coral bottom, maybe stuck in a cave, and, without a doubt, be gasping for air.

But all this takes quite a bit less energy, strength, and stamina than what's required to be successful. To campaign the Pipeline, or any big surf, calls for a conditioning level of 100 percent—anything less is dangerous. Just to surf on a regular basis demands total conditioning.

The dilemma is that often the waves aren't there when you have the time for surfing, so how do you stay in shape for whenever the surf does come up? You do other stuff like paddle boarding, yoga, swimming—anything it takes, because there's nothing worse than being weak when the waves are strong.

Surfing is 90 percent paddling. Fast paddling is more than a function of strength and stamina alone; it requires technique, rhythm, strategy, tactics, and most of all, absolute spontaneity. The surf zone is the ultimate fluid situation where something is always happening because everything's always moving.

To be able to meet the challenge of the surf requires much more than just a training program. Once you accept that challenge, what generally occurs is a total change of lifestyle. Once you're in the life you can only then begin to specialize your training and conditioning activities.

Surfing is the single most complete activity you can do—it combines an all-body exercise in the best environment possible to stimulate physical, mental, and especially spiritual well-being.

—Gerry Lopez set the standard by riding one of the world's most dangerous breaks, the Banzai Pipeline. Born and raised in Honolulu, Lopez represented the Hawaiian World Contest teams in 1970 and 1972. He won the Pipeline Masters twice and eventually would have the event named after him. Visit him at gerrylopezsurfboards.com

7

CREATING A WORKOUT
SCHEDULE

After reading about all the various stretches and exercises described in this book, you may be thinking, "So when am I going to have time to actually surf?!"

Relax—the one thing we definitely want to avoid is overtraining. Overtraining can lead to injury, and that means time out of the water. These workouts are designed to improve your surfing abilities, as well as your overall physical fitness. The trick is to figure out which workouts you can most benefit from and how to incorporate them into your life so that they complement your surf time, not compromise it.

Stretching can and should be done every day before you surf. In fact, the only exercise you should do other than a warm-up or light balance routine is stretching.

You don't want to tire yourself out with cardio or strength training before you paddle out!

Now let's consider the other workouts presented in the previous chapters:

- Cardio Beach Workout
- Cardio Pool Workout
- The Surf Flex Workout (Swiss Ball exercise)
- Dry Land Workout
- Wahine Workout

HOW DO YOU STAY IN TOP CONDITION FOR SURFING?

"I'm 43 and I've been surfing since I got my first styrofoam surfboard at age 6. There are four things I do to enhance my life and enable myself to keep surfing: aerobic fitness, upper body and abdominal strength training, flexibility training, and diet. In my opinion, these are the four most critical areas to maintain all year long to be able to surf well and enjoy life.

"For aerobic fitness and leg strength, I run three times per week, four to five miles per workout. For upper body strength I do push-ups and work out with dumbbells doing military presses and bicep and tricep curls. I also do lat pull-downs and upright rowing on Cybex machines twice per week, to mimic paddling. For abdominals I do at least 125 crunches daily, with twisting motion to exercise the obliques. These muscles are easy to forget but very important for a quick stand up on your board. For flexibility, I do static stretching every day—in the morning when I get up and at night before I go to bed, aiming particularly on my lower back, legs, and pelvic area.

"When I'm surfing regularly in the summer and fall the only exercise I continue to do is running because I find hours and hours in the water keeps my abs and paddling ability at a high level.

"Diet is the last area that I find has a great impact on my general health and overall agility, particularly as I get older. If I eat bad I feel bad, but for the past 23 years I've regulated my diet to contain lots of organic and unprocessed vegetables, fruits, some lean meat, soybean products, and fish. I avoid all foods containing hydrogenated oils, which are wicked on the body. (It hasn't been easy to avoid, since just about everything in mainstream food stores has this ingredient. Fortunately, Whole Foods Market is nearby, so I shop there exclusively.) Also, I don't eat fast food or drink sodas—too much trans-fatty acids, salt, and sugar in those menus. Also, I take daily supplements of antioxidants, ginseng, and ginger root, plus some other things, like green tea. I drink coffee only on weekends. I believe this has had a positive impact on my general health.

—Mark McMullen
President, The Longboard Network (www.longboard.net)

If you're surfing almost every day during the peak surf season, you may want to do the cardio workouts three or four times a week, but go light on the strength training workouts. Then, during the off season, you should start the Surf Flex Workout two or three times a week. To give yourself variety, substitute the Dry Land Workout once a week for the Surf Flex Workout. (Women should try to do the Wahine Workout once or twice a week in addition to the Surf Flex Workout.)

When strength training, it's important to remember to rest at least one day between workouts. In other words, never do strength training two days in a row unless you train different muscle groups. (Cardio training can be done more often.) Your muscles become stronger when they rest and repair after a workout, so by training too soon after a workout, you can actually injure yourself and impede the strength-building process. It's also a good idea to leave one day a week for rest—a day when you do no training.

Here is a sample workout schedule for the off season:

Monday:	Surf Flex Workout
Tuesday:	Cardio Beach Workout
Wednesday:	Dry Land Workout
	(plus Wahine Workout for women)
Thursday:	Cardio Pool Workout
Friday:	Surf Flex Workout
Saturday:	Cardio Beach Workout
Sunday:	Rest

Here is a sample schedule for the surf season:

Monday:	Surf, Cardio Beach Workout
Tuesday:	Surf, Surf Flex Workout
Wednesday:	Surf, Cardio Pool Workout
Thursday:	Surf, Surf Flex Workout
Friday:	Surf, Cardio Beach Workout
Saturday:	Surf
Sunday:	Rest

If you're lucky enough to live in an area where the surf season is all year (or if you are a competitive surfer), you should concentrate on strength training at the time of year when the waves are the weakest. This will help develop your strength and endurance for that big swell or contest.

Depending on your age and fitness level, when you start these workouts you may be able to do just one or two days a week of only one or two of the workouts—that's OK. Work at your own pace and you will see improvement, both in the number of workouts you can complete with more and more ease, as well as in the quality of your surfing— and that's the whole point!

SURF FLEX ASKS LAYNE BEACHLY:

HAVE YOU EVER OVERTRAINED?

"The best advice I received in regard to training for surfing came from Tom Carroll. He said, 'There is no better training for surfing than surfing.' Mind you, we were lifting weights together at the time in our coach's backyard, but Tom always made me go surfing with him afterwards to make sure my muscles stayed supple. (He is just an overgrown grommet who probably still surfs more than half the guys in the top 44.)

"Training differs dramatically for each individual, but if you want to be competitive you have to be prepared to go outside of your comfort zone to some extent, but not so far to the point of wearing yourself down. Like everything in life, moderation is the secret. I was so motivated by training that my health actually suffered. I ended up with chronic fatigue syndrome because I ignored the warning signs of my body asking me for a break that I didn't think was allowed or necessary. I have now learned how to balance my training between the gym and the ocean. But, if I am feeling tired or run down a surf will always make me feel much better than a good workout. Surfing everyday regardless of the conditions keeps my timing, technique, and energy levels in tune. Practice makes perfect."

—Layne Beachley, two-time ASP Woman's World Champion (1998, 1999), winning once by the highest point margin ever—2320 points. She has appeared on such national television programs as *60 Minutes*, the *Today Show*, and *Good Morning Australia*.

8

TOYS FOR BOYS & GIRLS

E xercise can get pretty boring, especially for surfers. There isn't much out there that can stimulate your nervous system like riding a wave. So finding fun and challenging alternatives to standard exercises is a terrific benefit. The two pieces of equipment used in the following pages will really charge up a surfer balance system. When doing exercises on a rocker board or a Dyna-Disc pillow, the core musculature instantly kicks in. Therefore, all the movements or exercises you do

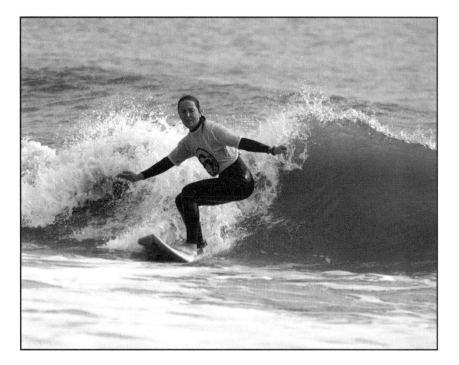

on these will emanate for your core (your lower back, abs, hips and thighs), known in sports as *the power zone.* Here are a few exercises to try, but have fun. Your imagination is your only limit!

A rocker board is a board with a rocker underneath. These are easy to make with a thick piece of plywood two feet wide and a wooden dole anywhere for one to three inches thick nailed underneath. The Dyna-Disc isn't as easy to make—unless your folks own a rubber factory. A Dyna-Disc is an air-filled disc 14 to 17 inches in diameter. Both the Dyna-Disc and the rocker board can be found at www.getfitnow.com.

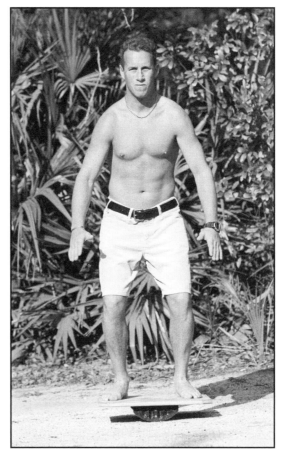

BALANCE AND ROCK

Stand on the rocker board and keep your knees slightly bent. Try to keep the edges of the board from touching the ground.

BALANCE AND SQUAT

Standing on the board, do 20 squats. Add intensity by holding weights in your hands. Focus on maintaining a flat back. Try to keep the edges of the board from touching the ground.

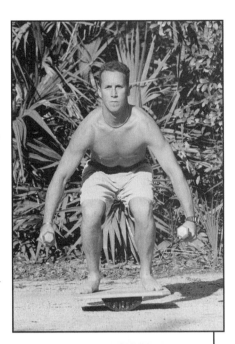

BALANCE, SQUAT, AND PRESS

Stand on the board with weights in your hands. Squat and press the weights over your head as you stand.

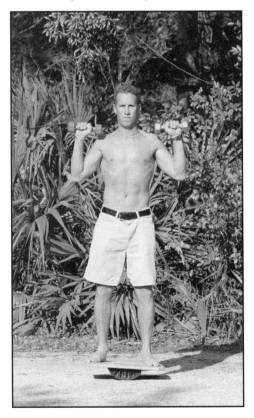

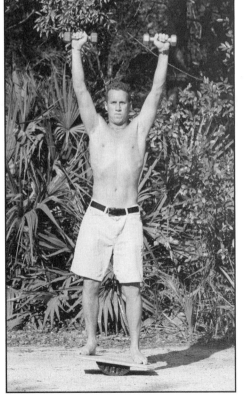

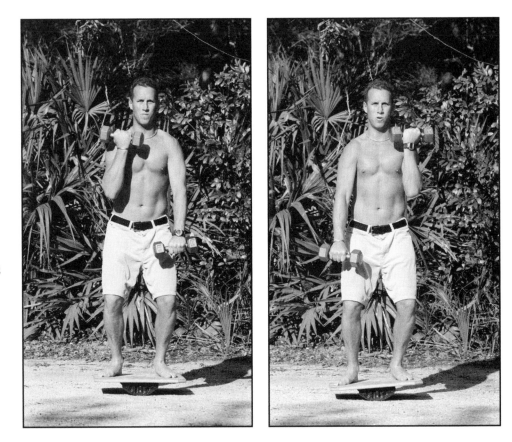

BALANCE AND CURL

Standing on the board, do 20 bicep curls, alternating hands. Notice how the body compensates to maintain balance as the weights in your hands alternate.

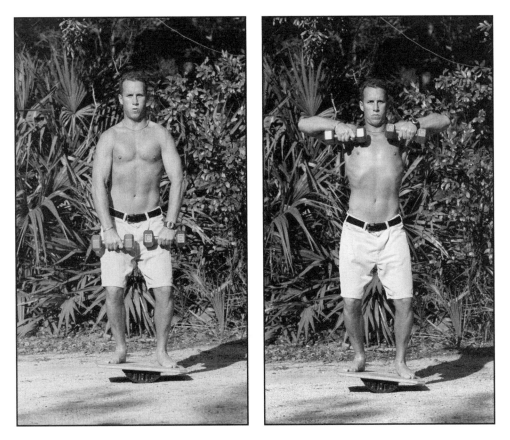

BALANCE AND UPRIGHT ROW

Hold the weights in your hands and keep your shoulders back. Lift the weights to chest-height. Try lifting the weights one at a time while maintaining your balance.

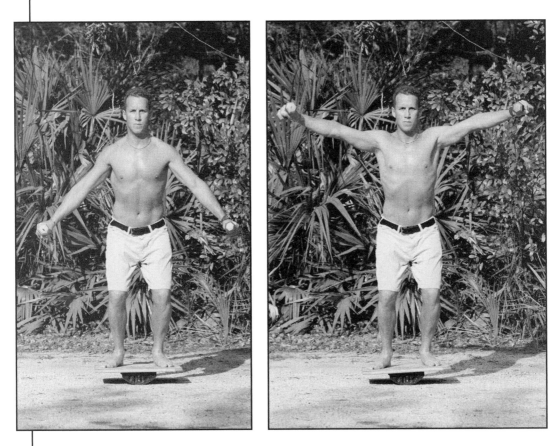

BALANCE AND LATERAL RAISES

Standing on the board, keep your elbows slightly bend as you lift the weights. For a more challenging move, lift one arm at a time.

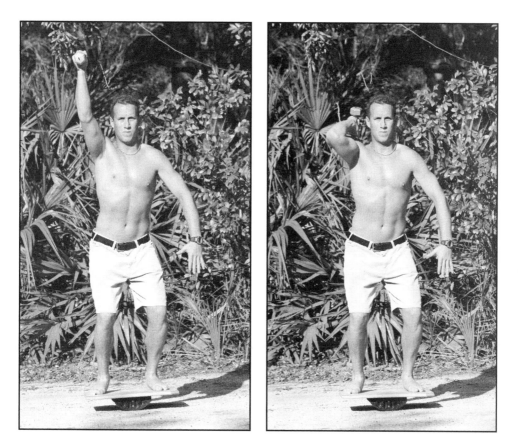

BALANCE AND EXTEND

Stand on the board and do 20 dumbbell tricep raises. This exercise is more challenging if both hands hold one weight overhead.

The Dyna-Disc can be a little more challenging than the rocker board. Whereas the rocker board moves from side to side, the Dyna-Disc requires you to maintain stability over 360 degrees.

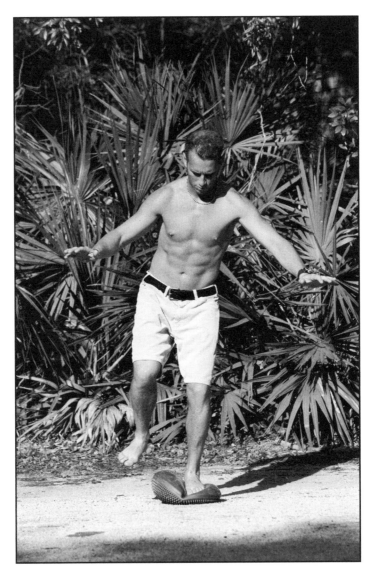

BALANCE AND SINGLE-LEG SQUAT

Stand on the Dyna-Disc and raise one leg. Try to maintain your balance. This will help train your ankle and foot muscles. Hold the position for one minute. You will begin to feel this exercise engage your gluteus (butt) muscles.

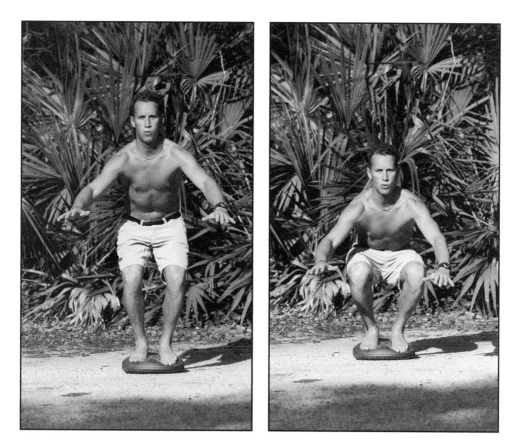

BALANCE AND SQUAT

Stand with both feet on the Dyna-Disc and do squats. This is very difficult, so don't be surprised if your legs shake when you do them for the first time. Keep doing them— you'll get better quickly. Do 10 reps. Observe your posture. If your chest is falling into your knees, modify your range of motion until your flexibility improves.

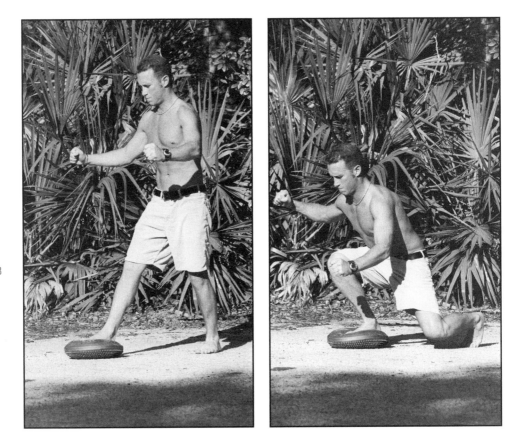

BALANCE AND LUNGE

Stand with both feet together, then lunge forward with one leg, placing your front foot on the Dyna-Disc. Push back to your original position, standing with both feet together. Alternate feet and repeat. This is an excellent exercise for strengthening and stabilizing the muscles, and helps develop balance.

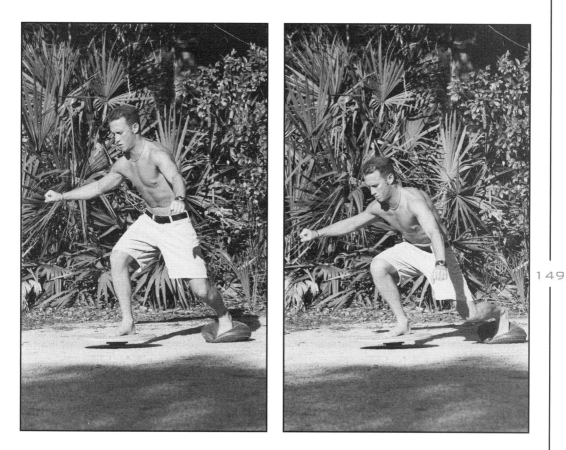

DISK AND ROCKER LUNGE

Now we're getting creative! Do 10 standing lunges with one foot on the rocker board one on the Dyna-Disc.

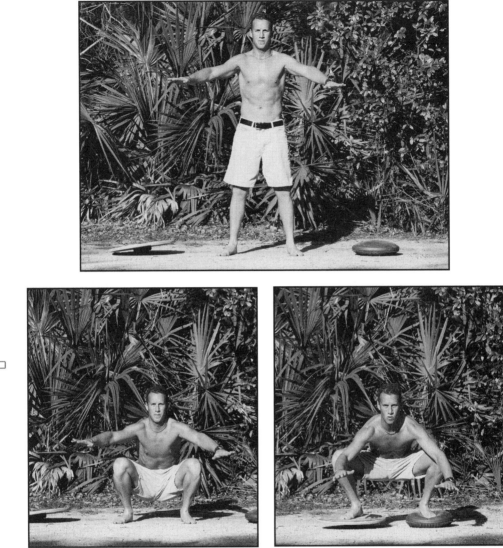

DISC AND ROCKER SQUAT

Place your feet approximately shoulder-width apart with one foot on the rocker board and the other on the Dyna-Disc. Do 10 squats. You can increase the intensity of this exercise by holding weights in your hands. Notice how my hero Buddy is leaning forward when he's squatting on the balance apparatuses. This ain't easy!

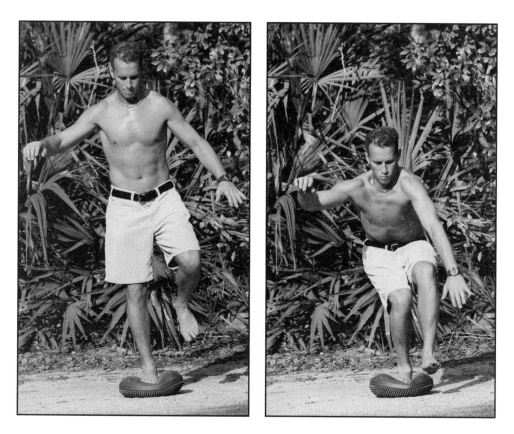

SINGLE-LEG SQUATS

This squat is an ultimate exercise in strength, stability and balance. Doing a few of these before hitting the surf will charge up your balance system. Try these with weights in your hands when doing a strength workout. Squat, then press the weights overhead as you straighten your legs.

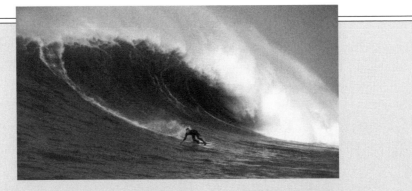

INJURIES AND INSIGHT by JEFF CLARK

"All this year I've been trying to manage the pain in my back. It got so bad that I had some x-ray's done and, when they found a fracture, I had an MRI done. This revealed a bulging disc between numbers 3 and 4 in the posterior vertebrae. Moving down to the bottom of my spine the doctors found a herniation. My routine this year has been very limited because of the overall discomfort. I spent as much time in the water as I could, but some days I could not even get to my feet. Off to the chiropractor, I went back to the stretching, but not so much that it would irritate the nagging injures. When I felt more flexible, I would get back in the water and paddle as hard as I could; this in turn would put me back in the pain management zone.

"When October 28 came around the waves were so big that I was not going to take a hit in the pit. The first thing I did was to feel out my board and see how far it could be pushed. Once I knew the limitations of my equipment I was ready to go. There was one stipulation—don't fall! The thing that I have going for me is my knowledge of the way a wave breaks at Mavericks at any size. My skill and knowledge and desire completely overcame what I lacked in conditioning. This is not something that one should rely on, however. For me, it was a hand that was dealt to me and I had to deal with it the best that I could. For me, that meant no mistakes as just one could cost me my life.

"This next year will be very different. Physical therapy is working and I have started to do more in the way of torso strengthening. My cardio capacity is the weakest that it has ever been. In the past I would ride the mountain every morning, followed by a yoga video workout. This gave me the leg strength and flexibility that surfing well requires. I found that the breathing exercises of yoga gave me calmness and clarity in extreme situations."

—Jeff Clark is the rider emeritus of mavericks and the director of the Quicksilver Men Who Ride Mountains Contest. Jeff Clark rode mavericks alone from 1975 to 1989 and was labeled one of the world's best big wave riders by *Surfer* magazine in 1994. www.maverickssurf.com

9

HELP YOUR RECOVERY WITH NUTRITION

G. Douglas Anderson, DC, DACBSP, CCN

hen a surfer is wounded or injured (including recovery from surgical procedures), the body has conditional increases in nutrients to facilitate proper and rapid healing. The following steps will create the internal environment necessary for recovery:

1. Drink extra water. Add a large glass as soon as you wake up in the morning, before lunch and before dinner.

2. Eat a high protein diet. Have at least three servings a day of foods such as fish, chicken, turkey, and low or nonfat dairy. Beef and pork are also good sources of protein but tend to be high in fat, therefore, use them in moderation. You can also acquire extra protein in your diet by using protein powder to make shakes and smoothies. This is especially recommended if you are a vegetarian. Use 25 to 40 grams of protein per drink.

3. Take a multivitamin, multimineral formula that provides you with at least 100 percent of RDA for all vitamins and minerals. Read labels carefully. If you use a one-pill-a-day formula, you will probably need to take additional calcium and magnesium. Other for-

mulas require that you take three or more pills a day to achieve amounts listed on the label.

4. Take extra vitamin C. During your recovery, multiply your body weight by ten and then round to the nearest 100 to find out how many milligrams of vitamin C you need per day. For example, 152 pounds x 10 = 1520, rounded to the nearest hundred = 1500 mg per day.

5. Do your best to stay away from junk food. Eating less junk food is always good to do but is especially important when you are recovering. Foods like soda, chips, candy, cake, pies, doughnuts, and cookies are low quality sources of calories. If you have a sweet tooth, try snacking on fresh fruits or sports bars such as Clif, Power, Balance, or Met-Rx. Ice cream lovers are advised to eat low or nonfat yogurt instead.

6. If you are on a weight loss diet put it on hold until you feel better. Increase the number of calories you eat to a level where you maintain your current weight. Trying to lose weight and recover at the same time will slow down the healing process. This, in turn, will inhibit your weight loss goals by extending the time you are unable to exercise and at the intensities required to burn body fat.

7. When you are better:

- Continue to drink plenty of water.
- Reduce your protein back to two servings a day unless you are involved in heavy athletics.
- Try to maintain healthy snacking habits.
- If you are on a weight loss program, resume it.
- Reduce your vitamin C intake to 500 mg per day.
- Continue to take your multivitamin at least five days per week.

A Diplomate of the American Board of Chiropractic Sports Physicians, Dr. Doug Andersen is a chiropractor and a Certified Clinical Nutritionist. He has published over 100 articles on nutrition and was a member of the ASP medical team from 1995 to 1999. He currently has a private practice in Brea, California and is the nutritionist for the Los Angeles Kings of the National Hockey League.

10

THE SURF DOC

PREVENTING AND TREATING
COMMON SURFING INJURIES

P roper stretching and strengthening exercises can help prevent a lot of common surfing-related injuries, such as pulled or torn muscles, knee sprains, and back pain. But such injuries inevitably occur, and most surfers tend to get right back up on their surfboards before their injuries have a chance to properly heal. To help you understand and treat common surf-related injuries and illnesses, I've asked Dr. Robert Budman (a.k.a. The Surf Doc on the Web at www.surflink.com) to prepare this chapter.

Dr. Budman discusses lower back pain, shoulder and knee injuries, sunburns, and travel-related medicine. In each section, he "fields" questions from actual surfers who've suffered from the ailment.

LOWER BACK PAIN

Have you ever "wrenched" your back while surfing? Perhaps you never actually fell, but the torque and muscle tightening during the rapid lip smack or kooky wipeout overloaded the soft tissues of your low back. These tissues could include muscles, ligaments, discs, and cartilage—

any of which became inflamed. Think of the pain as an internal tear of the muscles and ligaments causing inflammation.

I tore something in my back once while surfing an unreal winter swell in December 1986 in Virginia Beach, Virginia. I was immobilized for almost two months. Imagine trying to do ER medicine with that kind of back problem! It usually takes six to eight weeks for low-back injuries to heal. Surfing in cold water generally doesn't help, and returning to the water right away may only increase the damage.

All injuries, especially low back problems, take time to heal. Rest, stretching, ice and heat packs, medicines, spinal manipulations, massages, physical therapy, and possibly scans or injections all have some role in treating and evaluating back injuries. But nothing can replace time for injured tissues to heal. That seems to be the most frustrating part for most surfers. Patience is important. See a doctor you trust and work through your injury. As symptoms change, perhaps nerve injuries (sciatica, pinched nerves, entrapped nerves) need to be addressed or new methods of treatment need to be considered.

I tell my patients to limit themselves by the discomfort. In other words, if it hurts, then don't do it! The old adage "no pain, no gain" does not apply to the vast majority of people. If you give surfing a try after an injury, see how you feel, but if it is painful, then stop. Remember to stretch slowly and progressively before paddling out.

Always do slow, steady stretches before each surf session. Never stretch rapidly or "bounce" your body while stretching.

QUESTION FROM SURFER:

A few months ago, while backpacking in Mexico, I sprained my back. My front ribs hurt really bad, and the muscles felt tight around my middle back. It was a few months before I finally went to the chiropractor for some deep muscle treatment. I felt better for a while, but the tightness is back, along with numbness in my right arm every morning when I wake up and sometimes during the day. Do you think I could have done something to the nerves, and what should I do to help the pain?

ANSWER:

You need to get to a medical doctor right away. My chiropractor buddies send me patients when the possibility of pinched nerves exists. What this means is something in your spine is pushing on the nerve as it exits the spinal canal. You feel the pain or numbness in the portion of the body where that nerve sends its branches.

QUESTION:

About two-and-a-half weeks ago, I was drilled by my board, right on the hip bone. (You really don't want to know how it happened.) Besides my whole side turning Technicolor, it was very painful and limited normal movement for about a week. As one side got better, the other side became very stiff and achy. Now, right and left hip areas are better, but my lower back hurts. What did I do to myself?

ANSWER:

First, you sustained a contusion to the hip. That would be the physical damage done by the surfboard's hitting the hip. Then you developed a hematoma (the Technicolor part), a blood collection in the tissues where the damage occurred. When you favored one side because of pain, the other side had to compensate. These muscles became sore. Subsequently, the whole alignment of your body was out of sync, so the spinal region got sore as well. Ice and compression would have helped the original injury. Then stretching and manipulations could have helped the rest. Sometimes, injuries such as this take weeks to clear up, depending on the extent of damage and the adequacy of treatment. A chiropractor or physical therapist could certainly help you.

SHOULDER INJURIES

QUESTION:

About a week ago, I had a killer four-hour session, followed by hot pain in my shoulder whenever I tried to lift anything. Having had some experience with nagging tendonitis, I started icing and taking 600 mg. of Advil three to four times a day. That didn't help, so I went to the doctor, and after a full series of mobility tests he diagnosed it as bursitis. It hurts only when I raise my left arm up and away from my shoulder (like an "iron cross" pose) and then rotate the arm. There's lots of clicking and popping. I was given a cortisone injection, which seems to have helped, and I'm taking a few weeks off from surfing.

Do you recommend any exercises or specific pre-surf warm-ups to help mitigate or prevent reinjury when I get back in the water? I can guarantee that I'm getting wet again!

ANSWER:

Bursitis is a swelling or inflamed sac of fluid that allows tendons and muscles to move over and around bony surfaces and joints, particularly shoulders, elbows, hips, and knees. Sometimes these inflamed sacs have to be drained, for example in the case of "Popeye elbow," better known as olecranon bursitis. The other things you mentioned, like rest, ice, and ibuprofen can help mitigate, or lessen the severity, of the problem. I, too, frequently give cortisone injections for bursitis.

You should not neglect alternative treatments for these injuries either, such as chiropractics, massage, acupuncture, and physical therapy. Before a session, warm up and stretch for five to ten minutes. A trainer, chiropractor, or physical therapist can show you shoulder circles, wall climbs, and internal and external rotation maneuvers to stretch, strengthen, and increase the mobility of your shoulder.

Three famous shoulder exercises are wall walks, shoulder circles, and monkey scratches. Stand near a wall. Put your hand on the wall at shoulder height. Let your fingers walk your hand up the wall like a spider. That stretches the shoulder. For the circles, bend over and let your arm hang down. Make small slow circles in both clockwise and counter-clockwise directions. Add some weight as it feels better. Monkey's alternate between scratching the back of the head and the small of the back. That is a great rotational workout.

It sounds as though you may also have had a dislocated shoulder. Working out with light weights should rebuild the shoulder muscles and help prevent recurring problems. The muscles that cross a joint are the number-one stabilizers of that joint. So, with knee, ankle, and shoulder injuries, rehabilitation concentrates on strengthening the muscles around the joint. A physical therapist, chiropractor, fitness trainer, or doctor could give you some tips on proper conditioning techniques.

QUESTION:

While I was paddling out, two guys dropped in right in front of me. I tried to roll underwater but as I was trying this, a wave sucked me up and over. The wave took my board and my right arm over (backwards), yet didn't pay quite as much attention to the rest of me. Yes, it hurt, but I stayed out for a while, hoping that it was just a muscle thing. It got better slowly. If I traumatize the shoulder, it starts to hurt again. Did I dislocate it or separate it or what?

ANSWER:

If you dislocated it you would have felt it come out of socket and go back into place. My guess is that you hyperextended it or over rotated it. That can cause a severe sprain of the ligaments around the shoulder joint. When you stress the joint again, it can be painful. This can also lead to the dreaded condition called rotator cuff injury. The rotator cuff consists of 4 important muscles and their tendons that help to move the arm at the shoulder joint.

Ice and anti-inflammatory medication may help in the short run. In the long run, you need to exercise, stretch, and strengthen the joint. If you have recurring problems, get an orthopedic doctor's opinion. (Hint: Sometimes the surf docs at surf contests take a look at surfers' injuries for FREE! Also, some chiropractors may be there, and they can help you out too!)

An MRI (magnetic resonance imaging) is a great way to take a look at the joint without surgery to determine what types of problems might be occurring. Ultrasound can be a great way to image the shoulder, too. The problem might be partly due to aging or a genetic predisposition. Or you could have a spur on your shoulder. Spurs tend to be chronic. Surgery could remove the spur, but it might not relieve the pain, and it won't strengthen the shoulder. Many people experience resolution of discomfort despite the spur's remaining. Or you may have an inflamed or "worn down" bursa sac. Additional and/or alternative therapies would include steroid injections, ultrasound treatments, chiropractic intervention, acupuncture, and biomagnetics, just to name a few.

159

ABOUT THE SURF DOC

Robert D. Budman, M.D., is a board-certified family physician with over 20 years of surfing experience. He started surfing on the mid-Atlantic coast in Ocean City, Maryland, and completed his undergraduate studies at the University of Maryland with a B.S. in zoology. He did his medical training at the Medical University of South Carolina in Charleston. After a couple years of surfing the Carolina breaks, he did his initial residency training in

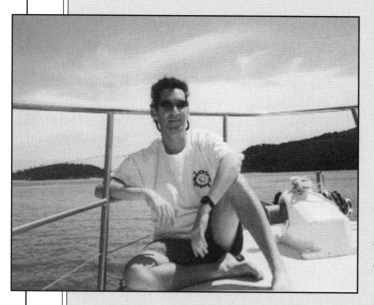

Norfolk, Virginia, where he especially enjoyed the Outer Banks and Hatteras surf breaks. Dr. Budman has surfed extensively throughout the United States, including Hawaii, as well as internationally. His other work includes cruise doctoring, Relief Doctor in the Australian Outback, and Expedition Physician for the 1998 Titanic Research and Recovery Expedition.

Based in Huntington Beach, California for the past several years, Dr. Budman is on staff at the University of California Irvine as an Associate Clinical Professor teaching Family Medicine as well as maintaining a busy private urgent care and travel medicine practice in Orange. He has treated a wide range of surf- and sports-related injuries. He still maintains an avid surfing appetite as well as a strong interest in human, environment, and ocean preservation (stemming from his zoology background). If, after reading this chapter, you'd like more information and injury-prevention tips, you can visit his Web site at www.surflink.com, or e-mail him at SurfLinkMD@aol.com.

The knee is the largest joint in the body. It is comprised of the femur (thigh bone) and tibia and fibula (leg bones). Important groups of muscles, like the quadriceps (thigh muscles) and hamstrings (muscles on the back side of the thigh) give the knee strength, stability, and of course its ability to move. Additionally, the knee has ligaments to hold the bones together and cartilage between the ends of the bones to provide a smooth surface for movement. Finally, the menisci aid in stabilizing the joint as it flexes, extends, and rotates.

The number of possible injuries to the joint are many, with all of these different structures involved. I advise anyone with knee pain to seek the advice of a specialist rather than trying to make his or her own diagnosis. It is even difficult for doctors to pinpoint the exact problem in many cases, and you may need x-rays, splints, crutches, drainage of fluid, medications, or perhaps even surgery to repair the damage.

Knee injuries are greatly reduced when the knee is strong. This is accomplished by muscle strengthening and proper rehabilitation in case of an injury. Good equipment can also prevent injury. (For example, if your snowboard boots or bindings are on wrong you could get hurt badly.)

161

Once an injury occurs first aid is crucial. Rescue the injured person immediately from a dangerous situation. Then immobilize the knee, apply ice and compression, and finally elevate the knee. A health care professional can tailor this treatment to the specific needs of the injury based on a thorough medical evaluation.

The more common injuries are muscles strains, ligament sprains and tears, cartilage tears, tendonitis, kneecap dislocations, fractures, and arthritis. With this many possibilities you can see the importance of having a doctor helping out with the care of knee problems.

Rehabilitation is a crucial part of treatment. After major surgery or even a minor sprain, every knee injury requires a particular regimen of recovery that may last from days to months. Specific exercises are necessary to increase the motion, strength, and stability of the knee joint. Only when the knee has met the rehabilitation goals should you return to surfing.

QUESTION:

I have first-degree tears of my LCL, MCL, ACL, and PCL (ligaments) in my left knee. Also, my medial and lateral miniscus have been trimmed. I know the condition of my knee because of the two arthroscopes performed on me. I love to surf when I get the chance, but because of my injuries I worry that I may not be able to walk later on in life. Should I stop surfing?

ANSWER:

I had a similar injury and had to have an ACL repair. I still surf as much as possible, and I am not concerned about being able to walk later—especially as long as I am surfing now!

The best medical help is the doctor you trust. Ask around your town for the orthopedist with experience at evaluating and treating your type of injury. There is some concern that knees with athletic and overuse damage might develop some form of arthritis later on. The statistics aren't clear.

162

QUESTION:

I've been able to feel fluid on my left kneecap for almost two weeks now. It does not cause me pain when I walk, but when I surf it gets sore. I can't point to any one incident that caused this, but it may have been due to my knee getting slammed during duck-diving. I would appreciate any advice you have—I'm hoping I don't need an MRI due to the cost.

ANSWER:

Not all knee injuries require an MRI. Have you had a doctor examine your knee? The fluid might be in a bursa (a small sac in the body that acts as a cushion for a tendon), or it might actually be in the knee joint. We call that an effusion, which is a collection of fluid in the knee joint comprised of various proteins, blood cells, and other components of body fluids. It can be caused by a single traumatic event or repeated minor injuries to the joint. Get it checked by someone with orthopedic experience—don't guess.

QUESTION:

At the same time I noticed the weather beginning to cool off, I noticed that my knee hurt a bit when I went running. Then it began to hurt when I walked, and when I tried to run I would lose feeling in my calf. Attempting to use the Stairmaster at the gym became impossible, and it hurts on occasion when I swim. I always stretch out and warm up extensively, but it doesn't help. I used to run competitively, so I'm sure that both my hips and knees have been injured at some point in time. I can stretch with no pain or problem. Is there the possibility of my knee giving out on me when I'm surfing? Could this be tendonitis? What should I do?

ANSWER:

Yes, you could have tendonitis. Or, you could have a condition called chondromalacia patella. Or you could have bursitis. Or you could have arthritis. I suggest a check-up with your local surf doc for an exam and possibly x-rays. Sometimes it is just a matter of time for these things to heal; other times it requires medications, treatments (heat, ice, ultrasound), exercise plans (specifically for the problem that is found with your knee), and possibly bracing or taping.

163

SUNBURN

You treat sunburn the same as you would any other burn. Cool cleansing is the first step. It stops the burning process and guards against infection. Then apply creme on a regular basis to moisturize the damaged skin. This will also alleviate the itching that comes along with the healing process. Aloe is okay along with the moisturizer, but by itself aloe is not necessarily better than creme alone, according to most scientific studies.

The key to skincare is don't get burned. In other words, an ounce of prevention is worth a pound of cure. In this case an ounce of waterproof sunblock can help prevent short-term burns and skin cancer later in life. The key to using sunblock is application liberally about 30 minutes before contact with water. This allows the blocking agent to dry and bind to the skin. Reapply often while out in the sun. There are some minor controversies regarding sunscreen terminology. My suggestion is to use at least an SPF factor 15 or higher of the water-proof variety. Learn not to burn!

HEALTH TIPS FOR TRAVELING SURFERS

I get a lot of questions regarding the health aspects of exotic surf travel. Nowadays, with surfers and extreme sports enthusiasts going to all parts of the globe, it is important to be conscious of not only the health concerns of the region, but the politics, culture, and customs of the region as well.

I practice travel medicine in my regular medical practice. I urge everyone who is planning a foreign adventure to check with his or her local medical authority prior to such a trip. The Centers for Disease Control and the State Department regularly issue and update travel advisories for the medical and political situations of every country on the planet—even when countries change their names or are near governmental collapse.

Here are the main points of travel medicine for surfers. First of all, check on all your immunizations. Sometimes a simple tetanus booster is all you need. For more exotic trips vaccines might include hepatitis A, hepatitis B, rabies, Japanese encephalitis, yellow fever, polio, plague, typhoid, measles/mumps/rubella, and cholera. The difference between getting a shot and not may be your life.

Second, malaria is a huge concern as many surf trips are to exotic, tropical beaches. These moist sea-level areas harbor mosquitoes that are more than likely to carry the malaria parasites. Malarial infection leads to intermittent high fevers, chills, headaches, muscle aches, and a generally horrible feeling overall. The fever breaks only to return regularly every two to three days. This is the number-one infectious disease killer in the world, and it is in virtually every tropical surf spot in the world. Notable exceptions are Hawaii and Australia (the last reports I saw on Tahiti and Fiji showed no reports of malaria either). Everywhere else go prepared! Take appropriate clothing (to cover arms and legs), netting for beds (as most bites occur dusk to dawn), and mosquito repellent that contains DEET. Ask your doctor for prescription medications to take for prevention. If you come back from a trip and feel miserable with a chronic, recurring fever, then get a malaria test. Preventing mosquito bites will also prevent a mosquito-borne illness called Dengue (Breakbone Fever). Yellow fever is also carried by mosquitoes.

Third, watch out for diarrheal illnesses like Montezuma's revenge. In Mexico this frequent illness is usually just one to four days of watery diarrhea caused by the toxins of a bacteria commonly found in the general drinking water. It is easily prevented by avoiding tap water, ice cubes, and substandard food preparation techniques. Remember to drink only bottled water and sodas. Pepto-Bismol is a standard treatment for this. Your doctor can prescribe antibiotics in severe cases.

More dangerous are some of the other forms of diarrhea that can be contracted in certain areas. These are especially possible in Third World, underdeveloped, and remote surf spots. Cholera is a severe

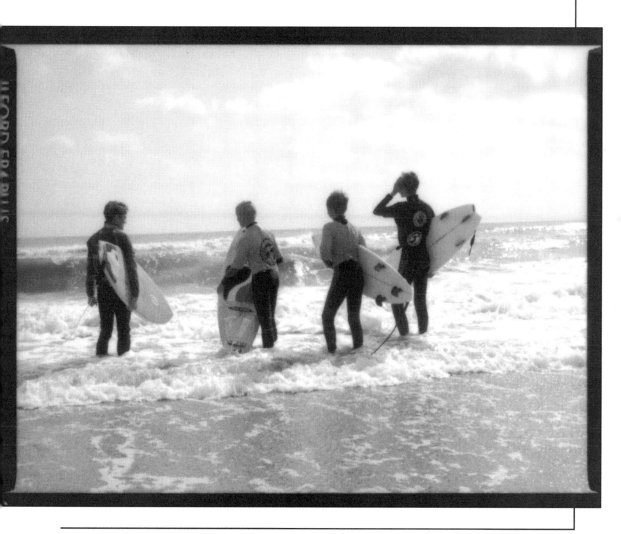

watery diarrhea that can rapidly dehydrate and kill you. Do not drink any ground water or even water from springs, showers, and sinks at Third World campgrounds. Treatment includes antibiotics and massive replenishment of fluids containing minerals and electrolytes taken by mouth (sort of like watered-down Gatorade®). Additional worries include amoebas, parasites like shistosomiasis, and a variety of dysentary (severe diarrhea). One article reported more than 20 known microbial causes of infectious diarrhea!

Other than the standard maps, surf mags, surf wax, and ding repair kits we all take on trips, don't forget some of the other essentials like tons of sunscreen, hats, and first-aid kits necessary for human ding repair! The contents of a basic first-aid kit vary. A few suggestions include bandages, antiseptics, antidiarrheals, motion sickness treatments, bug repellents, and sunscreen. And don't forget your regular prescription medicines if you are on any. In some cases it is advisable to carry copies of your medical history in case you have any problems on "surfari." Have fun and be safe.

SURF FLEX AND THE U. S. SURF TEAM

THE U.S. SURF TEAM AND SURF FLEX HIT THE BEACHES OF THE DOMINICAN REPUBLIC

Recently, *Surf Flex* author Paul Frediani was invited by Paul West to join The United States Amateur Surf Team in the Dominican Republic for the Encuentro 2000. As the U.S. Team's fitness and conditioning advisor, Paul Frediani introduced many of his flexibility and core strengthening programs to eager participants. Both the U.S. Team and the Dominican Republic Team welcomed the new ideas and concepts.

THE UNITED STATES SURFING FEDERATION

The United States Surfing Federation is a national organization dedicated to coordinating a competitive surfing program open to all levels of surfers nationwide. The USSF is committed to helping promote surfing and surfers in a positive manner on both a national and international level.

The United States Surfing Federation operates on a philosophy of teamwork. The organization has developed a strong foundation through the cooperation of its members at all levels, creating a balance of give and take so that all members, the USSF, and ultimately the sport of surfing benefit together. Our partner philosophy stands on this foundation. Cooperating and working as a unified team allows both parties to accomplish common and individual goals otherwise unattainable alone.

The United States Surfing Federation furthers its philosophy and goals through the collaborative efforts of its five member organizations, management, affiliated associations, and members of the Advisory Board. Each member participates in a team effort and continuously develops relationships with others who can help facilitate our philosophy and goals.

A BRIEF HISTORY OF THE USSF

The United States Surfing Federation was created in 1980 as the national governing body for competitive surfing within the United States. The International Surfing Association empowers the USSF to establish

and select members of the United States National Surfing Team repre-

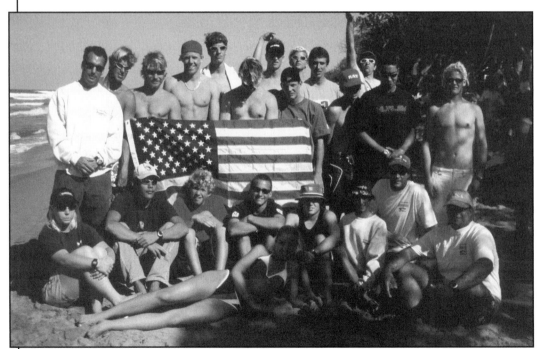

THE U.S. SURF TEAM, DOMINICAN REPUBLIC 2000. PHOTO BY CHAD OAKLEY.

senting America in all international competitions.

Now approaching the end of its second decade, the USSF continues to seek partnerships and opportunities that will help further the sport of surfing, its members, and their families, and broaden the market base for the surf industry. To ensure all team efforts are well focused and directed, the USSF is committed to:

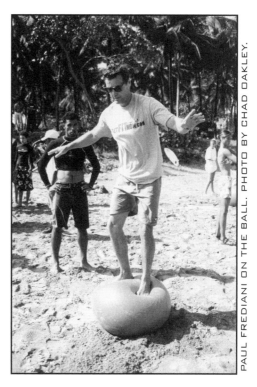

PAUL FREDIANI ON THE BALL. PHOTO BY CHAD OAKLEY.

- providing service, leadership, and a strong competitive foundation to its members as the highest priority;

- developing consistent, open communication with all other amateur and professional surfing organizations;

- encouraging a unified national competition program;

- promoting the acceptance of surfing in the United States as a legitimate competitive sport comparable to other mainstream sports already well exposed by the media;

- encouraging diversity by offering programs and competitions to surfers of all genders, races, ethnic backgrounds, disabilities, and abilities;

- supporting environmental issues;

- increasing beach access;

- forming scholarships and educational programs;

- providing medical and training opportunities.

Visit the USSF on the Internet at www.ussurf.org for more information, competition schedules, photos, and more!

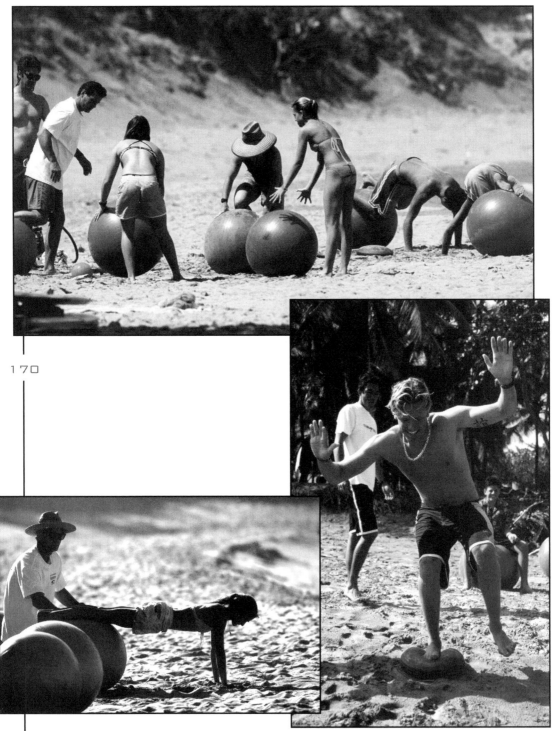

FUN WITH SURF FLEX IN THE DOMINICAN REPUBLIC. PHOTOS BY CHAD OAKLEY.

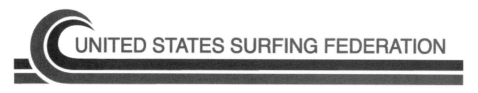

UNITED STATES SURFING FEDERATION

BECOME A MEMBER OF THE
UNITED STATES SURFING FEDERATION!

The United States Surfing Federation is a national organization dedicated to coordinating a competitive surfing program open to all levels of surfers nationwide. The USSF is committed to helping promote surfing and surfers in a positive manner on a national and international level.

To become a member, simply complete and return the form below and include your membership fee of $25.

[ ] Yes! I would like to become a member of the United States Surfing Federation. I am enclosing my $25 membership fee.

Name: _____

Address: _____

City: _____ State: _____ Zip: _____

Phone: _____

Area of interest: [ ] Competitive Surfer   [ ] Recreational Surfer

Would you like to volunteer for an event in your area? [ ] Yes   [ ] No

Mail your $25 membership fee to: United States Surfing Federation, P.O. Box 1070, Virginia Beach, VA 23451. Make your check or money order payable to The United States Surfing Federation.

VISIT THE USSF ON THE INTERNET AT:

WWW.USSURF.ORG.

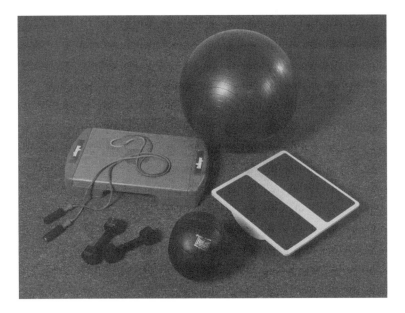